Praise for *The Fear Cure*

"Finally, a brilliant teacher from the medical community takes a

wonderfully up close and p ... *s been*
put to the test

— Larry Dossey, M.D., *Nev* ... *e Mind*

"The lives of a vast majority of humans are stressed with a panoply of psychological fears: fear of loneliness, fear of failure, fear of disease, and fear of judgment, among others. These chronic fears, which result in stress that undermines health and leads to disease and death, are responsible for up to 90 percent of all doctor visits. A valuable palliative to combat debilitating stress is provided in Dr. Lissa Rankin's new book, The Fear Cure. *This empowering compendium on the psychobiological impacts of fear offers highly effective personal management techniques to shift consciousness and transform chronic fear into health-enhancing behavior. For the health of civilization, I highly recommend Dr. Rankin's prescription for a positive drug-free healing experience that enhances intuition, integrity, and joy in life."*

— Bruce H. Lipton, Ph.D., cell biologist, best-selling author of
The Biology of Belief and *The Honeymoon Effect* and
co-author of *Spontaneous Evolution*

"An important book. It will change your life, as it changes the definitions of fear and courage. Learn to live. Learn to trust. Read this book."

— Sophy Burnham, *New York Times* best-selling author of *A Book of Angels*

"In a world fraught with risk and uncertainty, we could all use more courage. Dr. Lissa Rankin is the ideal guide—and this book is your anti-fear field manual."

— Chris Guillebeau, *New York Times* best-selling author of
The $100 Startup and *The Happiness of Pursuit*

"Dr. Lissa Rankin's book The Fear Cure *is just that, and more. This superb book shows you how to shift and transform your beliefs about your fears into new beliefs about your abilities to really feel your courage. You can then significantly expand and multiply your experiences of well BE-ing, grace, and goodness in every area of your life."*

— SARK (aka Susan Ariel Rainbow Kennedy), artist and author of
Glad No Matter What

"From the first page of The Fear Cure *I was drawn in, captivated by a subject matter that is so appropriate today. It seems that at every turn some aspect of our inner or outer world cries: 'Fear, fear, fear!' It is like the boy who cried wolf. Is there really a wolf? Or is it an illusion? In* The Fear Cure, *Dr. Lissa Rankin teaches us how to face our fear and shows us how to get to courage. Can you take the worst things that have ever happened to you and transform them into the best things that have ever happened to you? Dr. Lissa Rankin says 'Yes!' and then beautifully illuminates the path."*

— David Wolfe, author of *Longevity Now, Superfoods,*
and *The Color Cure* and founder of the nonprofit www.ftpf.org

The
FEAR
CURE

ALSO BY DR LISSA RANKIN

Mind Over Medicine*

What's Up Down There?

Encaustic Art

* Available from Hay House

Please visit:

Hay House UK: www.hayhouse.co.uk
Hay House USA: www.hayhouse.com®
Hay House Australia: www.hayhouse.com.au
Hay House South Africa: www.hayhouse.co.za
Hay House India: www.hayhouse.co.in

The FEAR CURE

Cultivating Courage as Medicine for the Body, Mind and Soul

DR LISSA RANKIN

HAY HOUSE

Carlsbad, California • New York City • London • Sydney
Johannesburg • Vancouver • Hong Kong • New Delhi

First published and distributed in the United Kingdom by:
Hay House UK Ltd, Astley House, 33 Notting Hill Gate, London W11 3JQ
Tel: +44 (0)20 3675 2450; Fax: +44 (0)20 3675 2451
www.hayhouse.co.uk

Published and distributed in the United States of America by:
Hay House Inc., PO Box 5100, Carlsbad, CA 92018-5100
Tel: (1) 760 431 7695 or (800) 654 5126
Fax: (1) 760 431 6948 or (800) 650 5115
www.hayhouse.com

Published and distributed in Australia by:
Hay House Australia Ltd, 18/36 Ralph St, Alexandria NSW 2015
Tel: (61) 2 9669 4299; Fax: (61) 2 9669 4144
www.hayhouse.com.au

Published and distributed in the Republic of South Africa by:
Hay House SA (Pty) Ltd, PO Box 990, Witkoppen 2068
Tel/Fax: (27) 11 467 8904
www.hayhouse.co.za

Published and distributed in India by:
Hay House Publishers India, Muskaan Complex, Plot No.3, B-2,
Vasant Kunj, New Delhi 110 070
Tel: (91) 11 4176 1620; Fax: (91) 11 4176 1630
www.hayhouse.co.in

Distributed in Canada by:
Raincoast Books, 2440 Viking Way, Richmond, B.C. V6V 1N2
Tel: (1) 604 448 7100; Fax: (1) 604 270 7161; www.raincoast.com

Copyright © 2015 by Dr Lissa Rankin

The moral rights of the author have been asserted.

Cover design: Elixir Design • *Interior design:* Riann Bender

The stories that appear in this book are based on real experiences.
Some of the stories are composites; some individual names and identifying
details have been changed.

'Endbeginnings', adapted from *Kitchen Table Wisdom: Stories That Heal* by
Rachel Naomi Remen, copyright © 1996 by Rachel Naomi Remen, M.D. Used by
permission of Riverhead Books, an imprint of Penguin Group (USA) LLC.

The information given in this book should not be treated as a substitute for professional medical advice; always consult a medical practitioner. Any use of information in this book is at the reader's discretion and risk. Neither the author nor
the publisher can be held responsible for any loss, claim or damage arising out of
the use, or misuse, of the suggestions made, the failure to take medical advice or
for any material on third party websites.

A catalogue record for this book is available from the British Library.

ISBN: 978-1-78180-399-8

Printed and bound in Great Britain by TJ International, Padstow, Cornwall.

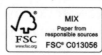

To April, whose brave is bigger than anyone I know

CONTENTS

FOREWORD

The Fear Cure is about wrestling with an angel. The angel is called Fear. The way to free yourself is to find the blessing that only this angel can give you. This book will help you find it and set you free to be fully alive.

I first heard the story of Jacob and the angel when I was very small. It was one of the many wisdom stories from Genesis told to me by my beloved grandfather, an Orthodox rabbi and a dedicated student of Kabbalah. As Grandfather told it, Jacob was traveling alone and as darkness fell he stopped to make his meal and sleep until daybreak. The place had seemed safe enough, but it was not so. In the darkness of the night he awoke to find himself gripped by muscular arms and pinned to the ground. It was so dark he could not see his attacker, but he could feel his strength. Jacob was a strong man himself and he struggled to be free, but his attacker was his equal and he could not free himself. They rolled over and over and wrestled on the ground the whole night long.

Eventually the night ended, and as the dawn came Jacob saw that he had been wrestling with an angel. With the dawn the angel loosened his grip on Jacob and tried to rise, but Jacob would not let him go. "Let me go," the angel told Jacob, "the Light has come." But Jacob held him tightly. "I will not let you go until you have given me your blessing," he said. The angel struggled but Jacob held him close. And so the angel gave Jacob his blessing.

As a little girl this made no sense to me at all. Jacob had struggled to be free all night long. Why not just let the angel go and run away? That's what I would have done. Besides, I loved angels. How could someone not tell the difference between an angel and an enemy? And even more puzzling, how could an enemy bless you? My questions made my grandfather laugh. "People confuse an angel with an enemy all the time," he told me. "Jacob does not let the angel go until he receives his blessing because the angel's blessing is what makes Jacob free."

It would be many years before I understood this story. At the time I held on to my fears tightly. I believed the only way to be safe was to be afraid.

My family actually cultivated fear in its children. After I was severely bitten by a stray dog and had to have a series of painful rabies shots, I became frightened of all animals. My parents encouraged my fear in the belief that it would keep me safe. As a result, my fear of animals grew so severe that it became a phobia.

I was 27 years old when I came to California to continue my medical training, and at first I lived with friends who had several small children and a big shepherd dog whose long yellow teeth terrified me. My friends tried to tell me that their dog was gentle and friendly, but I did not have the courage to face my fears. In the weeks that I was their houseguest, the entire family worked together to be sure that there was always a door between me and this dog. The dog roamed the house freely at night and I kept my bedroom door not only closed but locked.

One morning I awoke early with the need to use the bathroom. It was 6 A.M., too early for most of the family to be awake, so I was trapped in my bedroom by my fear. But perhaps someone else *was* up and about this early? Opening my door cautiously, I was relieved to hear four-year-old Bridget singing to herself in the living room. If I could reach her before the dog found me, she could put the dog outside. Despite my fear I tiptoed down the corridor and peered around the edge of the living-room door. But Bridget was not singing to herself. There was the shepherd lying on his stomach on the rug. Bridget in her little pink nightie was lying on the rug on her stomach too. She had a tube of toothpaste and a toothbrush and was brushing the dog's big teeth, all the while singing to him, "You'll wonder where the yellow went when you brush your teeth with Pepsodent." The shepherd's mouth was full of foam and he was wagging his tail so hard it thumped against the floor. I took a deep breath in and began to laugh.

In the blink of an eye I was free of a fear that had gripped me for more than 20 years. In that moment I knew that I was not afraid of the animals that lived in the world; I was only afraid of the animals that lived in my mind. My fear had not kept me safe from animals; it had only separated me from their love. Later, when I found my own apartment, I rescued a big orange tomcat. I have lived with a beloved animal companion ever since. That moment in the living room happened 50 years ago and I have been blessed by the angel every day since then.

Many of us who feel we do not have the courage to face our fears may have more courage than we know. If you have many fears, it takes courage just to talk to a stranger, just to answer the phone or go to the market to get bread. Just to speak aloud. Like a muscle that is used daily over and over, courage grows from being used like this. One day when you reach for your courage on purpose because something really matters to you, you may discover its power and its strength for the first time.

What you will also discover in reading *The Fear Cure* is that, surprisingly, courage is not the opposite of fear. The opposite of fear is joy. I had thought that joy was the same as happiness, but joy is far more durable than happiness. The capacity for joy seems to come from an unconditional relationship to life, a willingness to show up and meet with whatever is there. It is an openness that takes us beyond the wish to control life to the capacity to celebrate life. It moves us from an adversarial relationship toward life to the experience of mystery and wonder which is at the heart of life. Ultimately it can heal us.

There is in everyone a place beyond the preference for outcome, a place beyond a win/lose mentality and the fear that feeds on it. *The Fear Cure* offers us the option of trusting life itself and the realization that perhaps there is no way to lose except not to play. This wonderful book is about understanding and receiving the blessing in our fears, recognizing the power of our fears to guide us to our places of healing and free us to live with joy. There is no one alive who will not find a healing in it.

Rachel Naomi Remen, M.D.
New York Times best-selling author of *Kitchen Table Wisdom*
and *My Grandfather's Blessings*
Mill Valley, California, 2014

INTRODUCTION

Fear is only inverted faith; it is faith in evil instead of good.

— FLORENCE SCOVEL SHINN

When we drove into a tunnel on the way to a scenic overlook on Pikes Peak in Colorado Springs, my cousin Rebecca and I were feeling very Thelma and Louise in our top-down convertible with our long hair whipping in the summer wind. A short way into the tunnel, we noticed a stopped car blocking the road. Two men were standing behind the car, leaning into the trunk, as if the tire had blown and they were rummaging around for the spare. We braked and slowed to a crawl just as the two men did an about-face and came running toward us, wearing black knit ski masks and flashing shiny pistols. With the rag top down and no easy way to back out of the one-way tunnel, we were fully exposed, totally vulnerable, and trapped. Every cell in my body clenched as the masked men ran the few feet from their car to ours. My heart started pounding, and I could hear the blood rushing in my ears so loud that I almost couldn't hear their shouting voices screaming at us to give them our purses.

I felt terrified, but some other part of me took over in that moment. I was hyperaware of every nuance of the situation, simultaneously paying attention to the two masked gunmen, to where Rebecca was and how I sensed she was feeling, and to the sensations in my own body. Although I was frightened, there was a strange sense of calm as this . . . *something* took me over and guided me through the situation.

When one man asked me for my purse, the calm part of me watched me pull my purse out from under the seat and hand it over. My purse had little of value in it—a few dollar bills, some credit cards, a tube of lipstick. One of the muggers rummaged through my purse with his sausage fingers sporting a big gold ring. He pulled out my driver's license, shoving it in his pocket. He leaned so close to me that I could smell his boozy breath as he yanked the ponytail holder out of my hair and pulled out the silver barrette I was wearing, leaving my long hair covering my eyes.

I heard one guy bellow to Rebecca, "Get the fuck out of the car!" The calm part of me sent a mental message to her without speaking out loud: *Do as you're told and we won't get hurt.* But Rebecca was arguing with the man who was pocketing her camera.

"Can't I just keep the film?" she pleaded.

He repeated, "Get the fuck out of the car." From the corner of my eye I could see the shape of a gun held to her temple. At last she complied, taking her place next to me, our cheeks pressed against the chilly cement wall of the tunnel, our arms raised high.

Just then, I felt the cool barrel of a gun against the back of my skull. I stiffened, but the calm part of me whispered, *Just breathe. No sudden moves.* With the gun still pressed against my head, I heard the sound of a gunshot, and I felt my body quake. Electric jolts coursed through me, and my stomach turned. I didn't feel any pain, but I did feel warm liquid coursing down the side of my face. I wiped at it with my hand and looked at it, expecting to see the deep crimson I knew so well as a surgeon. But the wetness wasn't blood. It must have been sweat.

I assessed the situation, trying to sense with all five senses what was happening. I could smell the gunpowder. I could hear the footsteps on asphalt and the gruff breathing of our assailants. I listened for any other cars on the road but didn't hear any. I could sense Rebecca next to me, her energy even calmer than mine. The wind picked up and blew my hair into my eyes. I couldn't see anything, so my other senses were all heightened.

My mind quickly processed the gunshot. What had happened? If I hadn't been shot, had they shot Rebecca? In a wave of panic, I realized it would be worse to survive my closest friend's death than to be killed myself. Then Rebecca coughed, and I felt a rush of relief. We were both still alive.

Still wielding guns, the two masked men ordered us to turn around, step behind the convertible, and lie facedown on the hot asphalt. We did as we were told, and one of them yelled, "Now don't move!" Just then, I heard a smattering of gunshots and felt sharp rocks striking the backs of my bare calves. There was silence, then heavy breathing and a few muffled whispers I couldn't understand, followed by quick, thumping footsteps. Car doors opened and shut and, finally, an unmuffled engine revved and tires squealed. The car peeled out, and everything got quiet.

I lay there for what felt like a long time, my cheek still hot against the pavement, until I heard a car coming from the direction the gunmen had fled. The engine went silent. Two car doors opened and slammed shut. Then a man's soft voice said, "You two okay?"

I looked up to see two men in hiking clothes standing over us. "You ladies need any help?"

The danger was over . . .

WHEN FEAR IS YOUR FRIEND

What my body and mind experienced during the mugging was true fear—the kind of fear our bodies are hardwired to feel when our lives are in danger. My fear triggered the reaction that physiologist Walter Cannon at Harvard many decades ago named the "fight-or-flight" response, or "stress response," which is a healthy survival mechanism designed to put my body on full alert in case I needed to run away from my attackers or perform some Herculean act of strength that was necessary to save my life or

Rebecca's. When someone has a gun to your head, fear is something to welcome. It's there to protect you.

Without this kind of fear, you might walk right into oncoming traffic, befriend a rattlesnake, jump out of an airplane without a parachute, walk through a dangerous neighborhood at 2 A.M., or leave your baby unattended near a swimming pool. When appropriate stress responses are triggered, your body's natural survival mechanisms will help protect you and your loved ones. In this way, the right kind of fear can benefit your health. It can even save your life.

However, it's rare that life or limb is genuinely threatened. As prehistoric humans, we needed these primordial instincts much more often, given how vulnerable we were to predators, the elements, starvation, and disease. But things have changed. Few people reading this book are at risk of getting eaten by a tiger or starving to death. Most of the fears that plague us today exist only in our imagination. They are not real threats, but the amygdala in the primordial brain can't tell the difference, so the nervous system gets stuck in unnecessary stress responses. Our warning mechanisms malfunction, and we wind up feeling inappropriately afraid, which harms our health and leads to unnecessary suffering.

If fear can harm you and make you unhappy, you might assume that fear is something you need to get rid of. You might imagine you should add "Cure fear" to your list of New Year's resolutions, along with "Eat healthy" and "Exercise more." But that's not what I'll be suggesting in this book. Instead, I'd like to invite you to reframe your relationship with fear so fear can *cure you* instead.

Let that sink in for a moment. What if fear isn't something to avoid, resist, or feel shame about? What if, instead, fear is here to help you? What if fear is the finger pointing toward everything that stands between you and true well-being? Most of us devote a great deal of energy to organizing our entire lives around avoiding what we fear most. But fear can be a messenger that wakes you up to everything in your life that's still in need of healing. For example, if there's still a roof over your head and money in the bank but you're afraid of going broke, fear might be pointing to patterns you learned in childhood about financial lack. In order to experience the peace of abundance, you might need to address any limiting beliefs about money that keep you from thriving. If you're afraid of making yourself vulnerable and opening your heart to love, fear may be sending you a message about wounds from unhealed heartbreak in your past that need your tender, loving care. If you're afraid of getting sick, fear may be signaling you to stop giving so much and start prioritizing your own self-care. Fear carries with it a precious message, and if you're willing to listen to your fear, rather than run away from it, fear can help you get on the fast track to healing in body, mind, and soul.

In order to befriend fear, you have to know how to respond when fear rears up. When your life is in imminent danger, fear is meant to fuel you into action. But when what you fear exists only in your imagination, that's when you need to glean the message it is trying to deliver; otherwise the fear can take you over and drive your decisions. Transforming your relationship with fear requires discerning the difference between fear that points to real, present danger and fear that's trying to teach you about the blind spots and growth edges in your life. But how do you do this?

Psychologists schooled in the branch of psychotherapy called Acceptance and Commitment Therapy (ACT) differentiate between "clean pain" and "dirty pain." Clean pain results from real-life events—loss of a loved one, a broken heart, or injury, for example. Dirty pain results from the mental stories we create and judgments we make about our painful life events. For example, your boyfriend breaks up with you. This causes clean pain. Dirty pain follows when you make up a story about how you're not sexy enough or smart enough to be worthy of that guy who dumped you, and you then suffer from your self-judgment. Clean pain results when you break your leg playing baseball. Dirty pain results when you convince yourself you'll get kicked off the baseball team, lose your scholarship, never be able to play baseball again, and wind up worthless.

Feelings of fear divide along similar lines. I was originally inspired by this distinction to discuss what I planned to call "clean fear" and "dirty fear." But I was concerned that the term *dirty fear* might trigger feelings of shame in people who are hindered by this kind of feeling. There's no place for judgment in the process of letting fear cure you. Instead, we'll talk about "true fear" and "false fear" just so you're clear how to use the information fear gives you in order to fuel inspired action. True fear is the kind of fear that triggers necessary stress responses that protect you. True fear kicks in when life or limb is threatened, and it signals you to DO SOMETHING, pronto! True fear fuels actions that can save your life and help shield those you love from danger.

False fear, like dirty pain, exists only in your imagination. It's the voice that says your spouse is having an affair, when in fact there's no evidence—you're just primed to suspect it because your father cheated on your mother. It's your imagination prattling on that your boss is conspiring to fire you, when the truth is you just got a raise. It's the fear that nobody loves you and you're going to wind up all alone, when there's really a roomful of people who would do anything for you. It's the fear that you'll wind up a bag lady when, in present time, even if your bank account is dwindling, you can still pay the rent and put food on the table.

Every human on earth experiences both true and false fear, and both can help you. True fear protects you in a literal sense when you're in danger, or when someone you love is, but false fear can help you too, if you're willing to let it be your teacher. In this book, you'll discover how to unearth your natural courage so false fear can help you grow, rather than ruling your life, undermining your health, and robbing you of joy. Instead of taking your marching orders from false fear thoughts, you'll learn how to filter the messages of fear by letting the part of you I call your "Inner Pilot Light" translate.

YOUR INNER PILOT LIGHT

Your Inner Pilot Light is that ever-radiant, always-twinkling, 100 percent authentic divine spark that lies at the core of you. Call it your soul, your spirit, the real you, your Christ consciousness, your Buddha nature, your highest self, or your inner healer—this part of you is pure consciousness. The minute the very idea of you was ignited, this spark was lit, and it has been glowing away ever since.

Your Inner Pilot Light, which is the birthplace of courage, has the power to transform all the scary, courage-diminishing thoughts of your false fear into messages meant to heal you from your core. The voice of this wise part of you shows up as intuition, and unlike the thoughts fueled by false fear, it can always be trusted to guide your actions. When you learn to hear this voice and abide by its guidance, you become impossibly brave. In his book *Unlearning Back to God,* philosopher Mark Nepo describes this part of you beautifully as the original, incorruptible center of your self. He writes, "Each person is born with an unencumbered spot, free of expectation and regret, free of ambition and embarrassment, free of fear and worry; an umbilical spot of grace where we were each first touched by God. It is this spot of grace that issues peace."

You don't have to be religious or even particularly spiritual in order to align with the guidance of your Inner Pilot Light. You just have to be willing to remember the truth of who you really are. Your Inner Pilot Light never burns out, even at the darkest times of your life, but it can grow dim—and when you lose touch with this essential part of who you are, you're likely to let false fears run your life. When you're not tapped into your Inner Pilot Light, you can't hear the messages false fears are trying to give you, so it's impossible to let fear cure you. Instead, fear not only winds up making you unhappy, but as I'll prove to you later in this book, it can make you sick or even kill you.

This is what happened to me after I was held up at gunpoint.

HOW FALSE FEAR CAUSED ME TO SUFFER

After the incident in Colorado Springs, I had nightmares of looking over and seeing Rebecca on that black asphalt, lying in a pool of blood or feeling the gun pressed against my skull, hearing the shot, and feeling warm liquid coursing down my face that, when I touched it, stained my hand red. For over a year, I woke up multiple times during the night with my heart pounding, electric tingles zipping through me, and blood rushing in my ears.

On night call as an OB-GYN resident, I would be walking down the hospital hallway, pushing a patient on a gurney, and suddenly, with no obvious trigger, I would flash back to the scene. While my cognitive mind knew I was safe, my body flipped into panic mode. As a busy medical resident working 16-hour days, I didn't seek out professional help like I should have. Instead, I blundered through the aftermath of the holdup, which coincided with the dissolution of my marriage.

Before the Colorado Springs incident, I had already been burdened by countless fears. I was afraid of getting raped when I took public transportation to the hospital at 4 A.M. I was terrified of screwing up in the hospital and having someone die. I was scared of letting down my parents. I worried that I'd never be a good enough doctor. I was afraid of winding up alone after my divorce. I was even scared of roaches. I walked on eggshells to make sure nobody saw through the mask of perfection I wore in the hopes that others would love and accept me, in spite of my many flaws.

But after Colorado Springs, I was afraid of everything—the dark, loud noises, tunnels, scenic overlooks, convertibles, airplanes, strangers in the park, losing someone I love, daring to fall in love again. I was even afraid to talk to anyone about the panic that arose in the wake of the incident, afraid I would come across as weak, afraid it would hurt my professional reputation, afraid someone might prescribe Xanax and then I'd get hooked and wind up in rehab, or even worse, laced into a white straitjacket and locked away.

When I had a gun to my head, the fear I felt was true fear. My life really was in danger. But all the fears that followed were false. They existed only in my imagination, and none of the things I was afraid of ever came true. These false fears were trying desperately to shake me awake and show me the truth about the posttraumatic stress disorder I was experiencing. They were begging me to seek help, but I was still fast asleep back then, out of touch with my Inner Pilot Light and unaware of how fear could cure me, if only I was open to it. Instead, these false fears created so much unnecessary suffering in my life. With the cacophony of false fear voices screaming in my mind, I wound up feeling lost, disconnected, and at the mercy of a dangerous world.

It shouldn't have surprised me that in the midst of all this, during a routine physical my doctor noticed that my blood pressure was alarmingly high. A referral to a cardiologist revealed more pathology—a heart murmur, a cardiac arrhythmia, and even higher blood pressures. The cardiologist worked me up for other secondary causes of hypertension that might spike up my blood pressure—renal artery stenosis, an adrenal gland tumor, hyperthyroidism, Cushing's syndrome—but everything else came back normal.

The doctors diagnosed me with "essential chronic hypertension" and dosed me up on three drugs. But my blood pressure wasn't responding. My doctors told me my condition was chronic, that I'd have to take drugs for the rest of my life, and that I would likely die young of heart disease, given the severity of my high blood pressure and my youth at the time of diagnosis. None of my doctors ever once asked me what *else* was going on in my life, and because I had been brainwashed into the mind-body dissociation common in the medical establishment, it never occurred to me, either, to question whether my high blood pressure and heart conditions might be related to my countless fears.

It wasn't until almost 15 years later, when I was researching my book *Mind Over Medicine: Scientific Proof That You Can Heal Yourself,* that I fully understood how fear had hijacked not only my mind, but my body. I wasn't just suffering from the emotional and spiritual aftermath of what had happened in my personal and professional life, from the robbery to my divorce to the stress of my grueling job. My nervous system had been completely jacked up, and it was affecting every cell in my body through a complicated series of hormonal reactions that were making me sick.

Had I not woken up to the many ways that a repeatedly triggered stress response was contributing not just to my high blood pressure and cardiac issues, but also to a whole host of other health conditions that plagued me, I'd probably still be taking the seven medications doctors wound up prescribing for me. Fortunately, I did wake up. I began to understand how, if we're out of touch with our Inner Pilot Light, false fear leads us to deny what is true for ourselves, and how this betrayal of our personal integrity predisposes the body to disease. The shocking truth of what I learned flew in the face of everything I had been taught in 12 years of medical education—and sent me into an ego meltdown as everything I thought I knew about medicine was thrown into question.

THE PSYCHO-SPIRITUAL ROOTS OF ILLNESS

I didn't realize at the time that this shift in my awareness about what it really means to be "healthy" would not only transform my physical body; it would also thrust me onto a path of profound spiritual inquiry and discovery. While I am still very much a student of what makes the body wholly healthy, one thing I have realized after my own personal experience, as well as years of working with patients, is that it's futile to approach the prevention and treatment of disease without also learning to transform the false fears that predispose us to illness if we don't learn how to let them cure us.

While many physicians and other health care providers are also waking up to this truth, and while an increasing number of empowered patients are embracing the idea that fear and disease might be linked, this still seems radical to others within the medical establishment. Attention still focuses primarily on the biochemical causes of disease, without much consideration of the psycho-spiritual factors that have been proven to affect the body's biochemistry. While growing interest in the field of integrative medicine has raised awareness of the benefits of such health boosters as diet, exercise, natural alternatives to pharmaceuticals, complementary and alternative medicine, and stress management tools like meditation and yoga, far too little attention has been paid to the spiritual roots of disease and the diagnostic and treatment tools that have been employed by healers for millennia to tend to the health of the soul. This poorly explored area of medicine, where science and spirituality intersect, has become the object of my deep inquiry, both professionally and personally.

My passion for this aspect of medicine has not just fueled my own self-healing journey; it has also spawned Dr. Lissa Rankin's Whole Health Medicine Institute, a training program for physicians and other health care providers, which has included pioneering physician guest faculty such as Rachel Naomi Remen, Bernie Siegel, Larry Dossey, Christiane Northrup, Aviva Romm, Sara Gottfried, and Pamela Wible, as well as other revolutionaries including life coach Martha Beck, cell biologist Bruce Lipton, Whole Body Intelligence therapist Steve Sisgold, Mayan shaman Martín Prechtel, and movement medicine expert and Nia founder Debbie Rosas. Together, along with the visionary healers who participate in the program, we are on a mission to heal health care by reuniting medicine with its heart and soul, while inspiring patients to improve their health by finding the courage to let fear fuel growth, guided by the wisdom and courage of your Inner Pilot Light. When you let your Inner Pilot Light take the lead in your life, you not only free yourself from unnecessary suffering; you also pave the way for optimal health.

THE MASKS THAT FEAR WEARS

As long as fear lives in the shadows, hidden by shame, ignored out of ignorance, and unexamined by your Inner Pilot Light, it tends to poison you. You may not even be aware of how much fear influences your life. This is partly because, in our culture, fear tends to masquerade as a lot of other emotions. Perhaps because the word *stress* refers more to a physical reaction than to an emotion, we seem to be more willing to admit that *stress* is what plagues us, rather than worry, anxiety, or fear. In fact, for many, being stressed out is practically a badge of honor. We parade our stress as proof that we're busy, productive, valuable people leaving our mark on the world. But for many people, being "stressed out" is just code for being really, really scared.

When we're stressed at work, are we not actually just afraid? Afraid of making mistakes, of disappointing our bosses, of harming someone we're responsible for helping, of being perceived as "unprofessional," of speaking up for what we believe is right, of killing the patient / losing the case / failing to get the bid / letting the deal slip through our fingers? Aren't we afraid of getting passed over for the promotion, losing our relevance, getting demoted, being fired, and winding up unable to support the family? Aren't we afraid to demand shorter hours, ask if we can take time off work to attend school plays and soccer games, and insist that self-care is as valuable as work? Don't we fear admitting we're burned out and need a sabbatical, or setting boundaries with those we work with by unplugging from e-mail on weekends or turning off our cell phones after hours? Aren't we terrified others will discover that we're vulnerable and imperfect, when we expend so much energy trying to prove that we're professional superheroes?

Many of us wear work stress as the most acceptable badge of honor, but we also liberally admit that relationships are stressful. Parents are stressed with the kids. Spouses are stressed by each other. We're stressed out about whether to get married or have kids or break up, and we're really stressed when we're hopelessly in love with someone who doesn't love us back.

But what do we really mean when we say relationships are stressful? Don't we mean that we're afraid our loved ones won't stick around if they find out who we really are? Aren't we truly afraid of betrayal, rejection, infidelity, divorce, getting our hearts broken, losing the ones we love, or winding up alone? Aren't we afraid to admit that we want more affection, more connection, more help with the kids, less criticism, less judgment, more time, more sex, more space, more freedom? Don't we fear the vulnerability of fully opening our hearts—and the abject loneliness if we don't?

We're stressed about money, too, but money is just a piece of paper that sits in the bank. Aren't we really afraid of the loss of power, comfort, and safety we think money provides? Aren't we afraid we won't be able to pay the rent, get food on the table, keep a car, or cover our health care costs? Don't we fear being unable to save money for our children's education or fund our own retirement? Aren't we afraid we won't have enough of a safety net, should life's uncertainties thwack us upside the head like a cosmic two-by-four?

Even shame can be a mask for fear. When we feel shame—about our failures, our bodies, our sexuality, our addictions, our parenting styles, how we show up at work—what we're really feeling is fear: fear of being "outed" as imperfect, fear of rejection, fear of not deserving the love and belonging we all crave. Just as we hide our fear under the veil of "stress," we hide our shame in the shroud of arrogance, judgment, and contempt. But underneath our grown-up masks, we all have within us a frightened little kid, afraid that nobody will accept us for who we really are.

Fear can be sneaky, showing up in a variety of disguises that leave you unaware of how it's ruling your life. Many people feel uncomfortable even admitting that fear is causing problems. We see it as a weakness, something we should hide from others and overcome by ourselves. But this couldn't be further from the truth. True fear is a natural survival mechanism, here to protect you, and false fear is an important teaching tool, here to enlighten you. Fear affects every one of us. It's nothing to hide. On the contrary, it is worth examining so it can point you toward a better way to live, a way that aligns you with your natural courage and supports you in optimal health.

THE ROAD TO COURAGE

What is courage, anyway? Dictionary.com defines courage as "the quality of mind or spirit that enables a person to face difficulty, danger, pain, etc., without fear." But courage is not about being "fearless." Some of the most celebrated heroes and heroines have stood quaking in their fuzzy slippers while engaging in acts of wild courage. The Merriam-Webster dictionary defines it as "the ability to do something that you know is difficult or dangerous." But while the ability to do difficult, dangerous things may require courage, sometimes it's more courageous to avoid difficult, dangerous actions.

In spite of what Hollywood might lead you to believe, courage is not necessarily glamorous or sexy. It doesn't require fanfare or uniforms or medals or adoring fans cheering in the stands. It's not about weapons or car chases or daring stunts. Sometimes courage is an internal journey you take on your own—and everyone's journey is different. For some, just getting out of bed in the morning is unspeakably brave.

Courage is not about being reckless. It's not the daredevil parachuting off a cliff when there are sharp rocks below or walking a tightrope between two skyscrapers in the middle of a tornado. It's not the single woman walking into a dark alley at night when her intuition screams that she's at risk of being raped. It's not the single mother of four who quits her less-than-ideal job and winds up unable to feed the kids. It's not about getting into a ring with a bull that's out to make you into a horn ornament.

Courage is also not about doing something scary just because someone else pressures you to do so. It's not the soldier shouldering his gun and following orders that compromise his personal integrity. It's not the stockbroker who ignores his instincts and invests all his client's money in a risky venture because his boss thinks he should. It's not the gang initiate who holds up a bank teller, or the drug dealer who sneaks ten pounds of cocaine across the border for the mob boss, or the teenager who tries to ski a black diamond tree run just because his buddies tell him he's a pussy if he doesn't.

Courage is not about oversharing your vulnerabilities or indiscriminately exposing your heart. It's not the guy who keeps professing his undying love to women he barely knows. It's not the blogger who writes about her eating disorder, her drug addiction, and her romantic exploits, not because she's hoping to make others feel less alone, but because she's hurting inside and seeking attention in all the wrong places. It's not the woman who overshares details about her childhood sexual abuse as a way to jump-start intimacy. It's not the reality TV star who invites cameras into his bedroom while he fights with his wife in front of a million people.

It's not the bullied child who grows up and opens fire on those who bullied him. It's not the abused wife who stabs her husband in his sleep.

Then what *do* we mean when we talk about cultivating courage? Here's how I define it:

Courage is not about being fearless; it's about letting fear transform you so you come into right relationship with uncertainty, make peace with impermanence, and wake up to who you really are.

This kind of courage helps you make choices that strengthen rather than diminish you. Instead of allowing your choices to be ruled by false fear and the emotions that ride shotgun with it— anger, resentment, hatred, intolerance, depression, anxiety, and unresolved grief—courage stems from inner peace, and it empowers you to live in alignment with your soul's values.

WHAT INSPIRED THIS BOOK?

I researched and wrote my last book, *Mind Over Medicine,* because I was inspired by the brave patients who were willing to look at the root causes of their illness, write The Prescription for their own care, and make their bodies ripe for miracles. With many of these patients who made life changes that reduced stress responses in their bodies, thereby activating the body's natural self-healing mechanisms, I was blessed to witness spontaneous remissions. But in other patients, I observed a more concerning pattern. Some of my patients seemed so stuck in fear-based reactivity that they were paralyzed into inaction and couldn't make the changes they knew they needed to make in order to optimize their health. It was as if their souls got stuck inside cages locked by fear, and they spent much of their time and energy shoring up the bars of the soul cage so danger couldn't get in. What they didn't realize is that the soul yearns to be free of cages, and the very thing that locks us in the soul cage prison in the first place—fear—can be the key to let us out. For these patients, getting imprisoned by fear not only prevented them from embarking upon a self-healing journey; it also seemed to make them sicker.

I became curious as to whether there was scientific data linking fear to disease, and when I began researching it, I was shocked by the voluminous data proving without a doubt that the two are linked. Then I felt stuck. If fear predisposes the body to illness and I was going to shine a light on this truth, surely I couldn't just leave people more frightened without offering solutions. I knew that if I was going to share this data about the link between fear and disease, I also needed to offer hope for relief from fear's grip. And who was I to do this? I am a medical doctor, not a therapist or a psychologist, and while I often write about spiritual matters, I have no formal training that qualifies me to teach about them.

I tried to talk myself out of writing this book, but I was haunted by the data indicating that fear is one of the leading predisposing factors of disease in our culture. If fear could be argued to be as much of a health risk as a poor diet or smoking, as a doctor, wasn't it my responsibility to help patients address this very real health problem? What ensued was a deep dive into the body of knowledge about fear and courage, not as an expert, but as a curious student interested in doing whatever I could to counterbalance the disease-inducing ravages of fear with courage-cultivating solutions.

In the process of researching this book, I read hundreds of academic articles about fear in the mainstream psychology literature. I also read dozens of popular books about fear. Some, like *Feel the Fear and Do It Anyway* by Susan Jeffers and *The Dance of Fear* by Harriet Lerner, address fear from the psychological perspective, offering up practical fear-freeing tips. Others, like *The Gift of Fear* by Gavin de Becker, make the case for why fear is good for you, how it protects you from predatory criminals and life-threateningly dangerous situations. Still others, such as Pema Chodron's *The Places that Scare You*, Adyashanti's *Falling into Grace*, Michael Singer's *The Untethered Soul*, and Marianne Williamson's *A Return to Love*, address fear from a spiritual perspective.

I researched books and articles written about what helps us be brave, such as Brené Brown's *Daring Greatly*, Debbie Ford's *Courage*,

Ellen Bass and Laura Davis's *The Courage to Heal,* and Elizabeth Lesser's *Broken Open.* I also read a panoply of books addressing specific psychiatric conditions associated with fear and anxiety, including phobias, post-traumatic stress disorder, and generalized anxiety disorder. I even read a handful of memoirs, such as Elizabeth Gilbert's *Eat, Pray, Love* and Cheryl Strayed's *Wild,* written by people who overcame a fear-driven life in order to make courageous choices. In addition to reading a library's worth of academic articles and books, I also interviewed over a hundred individuals about how they overcame fear and chose courage instead, and I became fascinated (okay, *obsessed*) with what makes one individual resilient and brave while another gets trapped in a fear-based existence.

I realized that fear lives deep in the shadows for most people. We try not to talk about it. We certainly don't cop to most of our deepest fears in mixed company. Talking about fear at a dinner party isn't likely to make you popular. Yet we all struggle with it. As I interviewed more and more people about how they faced their fears and made brave choices in spite of them, I marveled at the ways in which different people handle adversity. Most of us do everything we can to avoid situations we don't want—divorce, the death of a loved one, bankruptcy, a cancer diagnosis, sexual abuse—and yet, time and time again, the most courageous people I interviewed told me that these events were the best thing that ever happened to them. I was baffled. How could such traumas be cast in such a positive light? And why were these particular people transformed in a deeply meaningful way when others experiencing similar adversity lost their spirit and shut down? Why were some people driven to protect themselves so fiercely that they wound up living only half a life, while others let fear act as the key that unlocked the soul cage? Most importantly, what might we learn from those who arose from the ashes and made the choice to live courageous lives? How might we unlock the soul cage ourselves?

I realized that fear can be a blessing, not only because it can protect you from danger, but because it can wake you up. If we can stay awake in the midst of scary, uncertain life experiences, the blinders that keep us from seeing our lives clearly may be lifted, and we may be blessed to know the truth about ourselves, how the world works, and why we are here. Fear points a bony finger at everything that needs to be healed in our lives, and if we're brave enough to heal it, courage blossoms and peace is the prize. As Christopher Hansard wrote in *The Tibetan Art of Serenity*, "Fear is just unrealized serenity." That's why The Fear Cure is not so much about curing fear; it's more about letting fear cure you.

But how does this happen? If fear leads one person to contract while another expands, what lessons or practices can we adopt that will help fear be medicine rather than poison? Is there something we can call upon when fear is gripping us, not just as a way to protect our health, but as a way to live more authentically, more soulfully, and with more joy?

What I concluded after all of my research is that there is no single "one size fits all" prescription that will help fear liberate you, rather than locking you in a soul cage. For one person, therapy is the solution. For another, it's a monthlong silent retreat or a pilgrimage. The prescription may be belly dancing or skydiving or signing up for an art class. It may be the practice of meditation, prayer, or EFT. Some people will require all of the above. One thing all the courageous individuals I interviewed shared in common was the ability to hear, interpret, and act upon guidance from their Inner Pilot Lights. Those unmistakable voices prescribed what they needed in order to let fear catalyze growth, and they were committed enough to listen and follow through.

The courageous steps the Inner Pilot Light prescribes to let fear cure you are outer actions that facilitate an inner process, because at its root, The Fear Cure is an inside job. It is about coming into right relationship with uncertainty and making peace with impermanence. This requires a shift in consciousness as you move from identifying with your limited self-image and its thoughts, beliefs, and feelings to fully realizing your unlimited true nature. The purpose of this book is to help you learn how to free yourself by making this shift. Ultimately, The Fear Cure is a journey of transformation, and it's yours to take, if you're ready and willing.

HOW TO USE THIS BOOK

This book consists of three parts meant to speak to different parts of you. Part One delivers a message to your cognitive mind, in case you're the kind of person who gets motivated by scientific evidence, that fear is not just a painful emotion that exists in your mind and makes you unhappy, but a life-threatening force that lives in the cells of your body and has the power to kill you. In the first chapter of Part One, I'll share with you the neuroscience and physiology of fear, explaining the mechanism of how a fearful thought translates into physiologic changes throughout the body. We'll also discuss how your nervous system can get hijacked by fear and trauma in such a way that stress responses are triggered automatically, bypassing the cognitive mind and hooking right into the limbic system, leading to phobias, post-traumatic stress, and other psychological disorders that may require professional help to overcome.

In the second chapter of Part One, I'll walk you through all the scientific data proving that fear increases your risk of almost every disease, especially the modern world's number one killer—heart disease. You'll discover that fear decreases your longevity and leads to physical suffering if left unchecked. The data I'll be presenting to you in Part One is not meant to scare you more; it's meant to educate and empower you, putting responsibility for your health back into your own hands, rather than leaving you feeling helpless, at the mercy of forces you think you can't control. Knowing how unchecked fear predisposes you to disease can motivate you to make healthy choices about how you might transform fear into medicine for the body, mind, and soul.

While Part One is intended to satisfy your cognitive mind's need to understand why you should stop letting false fear run your life and start letting it transform you instead, Part Two speaks not to your cognitive mind, but to your intuition, showing you that there's another way to live, and it's within your power to begin to live this way. In Part Two, we'll move from science toward the realm of spirituality, exploring where the two intersect. You'll learn the Four Fearful Assumptions, four limiting beliefs that lie at the root of many false fears. We'll discuss how to turn those four limiting beliefs around into the Four Courage-Cultivating Truths. At the end of each chapter in Part Two, you'll be given Courage-Cultivating Exercises intended to help you put these truths into practice in daily life. When you shift your worldview away from the common cultural worldview that's dominated by the Four Fearful Assumptions, trading them out for the Four Courage-Cultivating Truths, you pave the way for coming into right relationship with uncertainty and developing a healthy relationship with loss, such that uncertainty is full of possibility and loss can be the gateway to growth. Therein lies the real medicine.

In Part Three, you will be invited to marry your cognitive mind with your intuition so you can make this journey of transformation personal. You'll be creating your own Fear Cure, mapping your own courage-cultivating path, learning the Six Steps to Cultivating Courage, and letting your Inner Pilot Light write your Prescription for Courage so you can start blessing the world with your luminous light.

What's important to understand is that there are many paths to such freedom. Western psychology offers one approach. Eastern philosophies offer another. *A Course in Miracles* employs its own methods. Organized religions all offer their own faith-based guidelines for how to "fear not." Although this book is not in any way about any specific organized religion, I will draw upon some of the fear solutions offered by religious traditions such as the Christian mystics, the Jewish mystical branch of Kabbalah, the Islamic mystical branch of Sufism, Buddhism, and the Hindu tradition of yoga. All of these approaches are valid, and any of them might wind up being part of your own Prescription for Courage.

This process isn't a quick fix; it's a spiritual journey that requires time, practice, commitment, support, courage, faith, and radical acts of compassion, both for yourself and for the other fearful beings you encounter on your way. But what it offers is not a mere Band-Aid; it's real healing. By the end of the book, you'll discover that you've always had within you all that you need in order to look beyond your fear and find your brave.

WHY IT'S WORTH THE JOURNEY

If you've faced adversity in your life—and let's face it, who hasn't?—fear may have disconnected you from the voice of your Inner Pilot Light, causing you to compromise the integrity of your true self. These "sellouts" may be big, or they may be subtle, but over time, they grind away at the soul like sandpaper. Maybe, as I was, you're in medicine and you're asked to see 40 patients a day when you know that to be a true healer, you need more time. Maybe you're in advertising and you're asked to try to sell a product you don't fully support. Maybe you're a teacher and you're not allowed to hug the child you know just needs to be held. Maybe you're a banker and the powers that be won't let you lend the money to the small business owner who is going to lose his business if he doesn't get the loan you *just know* he'll pay back. Maybe you're a lawyer asked to defend the client with the most money, rather than standing up for what's fair. Maybe you're the politician who got into politics to be the voice for the people, only now you've sold out to special interests because you can't help the people unless you get reelected.

Maybe it's not about your job. Maybe you didn't speak up when someone was excluded from your social group because she didn't wear the right shoes or drive the right car, even though her heart was pure. Maybe you stayed silent on the church committee when they started talking about why they didn't want a gay preacher. Maybe you didn't stand up for your own needs when you were asked to sacrifice your own self-care for your family. Maybe you said yes when your Inner Pilot Light begged you to say NO.

Every day, your integrity is tested in a thousand ways, and every day, you have a choice. Fear will dish up all kinds of arguments for selling out. It will rationalize that you need security, safety, certainty, acceptance, and a paycheck. But what price are you paying when you systematically betray your truth, day after day after day? In this way, fear can be a blessing because it is always pointing toward those slips in integrity that need to be addressed. Even if the sellouts are subtle, and you're barely aware of what you're doing, compromise your integrity enough and your

Inner Pilot Light starts to grow dim. It becomes harder and harder to hear its guiding voice. Every time you betray your true self, a little piece of you withers away, taking with it your health, vitality, and happiness.

When you commit to aligning with your Inner Pilot Light 100 percent of the time, you're asked to do challenging, scary things. People you love may not support you, because you're no longer ruled by the fears most people use to control one another, and your new unpredictability makes them wary. You may start to trigger reactions in others, especially the ones who have rationalized why they're selling out their own truth every day. You become a mirror that those who sell out can't stand to look in.

But the ones who long to live in alignment with their own Inner Pilot Lights start flocking to you. Your changing vibration attracts your true soul community to you. And as a sort of thank-you for aligning with your true self, the Universe often draws into your life more and more true joy, unconditional love, professional vitality, physical health, and a sense of connection with the Divine. You may lose some, or much, of what makes up your comfort zone. But what you'll gain when you commit to this journey is *priceless*. The prize for your commitment is FREEDOM.

Are you willing to let fear cure you and explore how courageous you really are?

I dare you.

PART ONE

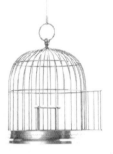

HOW
FEAR MAKES
YOU SICK

CHAPTER 1

The *The* PHYSIOLOGY *of* FEAR

The only thing we have to fear is fear itself.

— FRANKLIN D. ROOSEVELT

Eight-year-old April heard glass shattering down the hall of the single-wide trailer. She knew it was just the beginning of yet another one of those nights when Mom got out of control, as did the men she liked to drink with. April tried to run away, out into the woods in front of her house. But her lungs clamped down, and she was so short of breath before she even started running that she knew she had already lost this fight. The next thing she knew, a strange man was coming toward her, and her body was wracked with indescribable pain.

April doesn't remember anything else from that night. But she does remember that, soon afterward, her mother vanished. No explanation. No apologies. No good-bye. April tried to convince her little brother that their mother wasn't ever coming back, but he stood at the back of the couch and watched the door for weeks.

After her mother walked out, fear began to dominate April's life even more. She stopped trusting even close friends and social workers who tried to help. She lay awake at night, terrified that one day someone would take her away and separate her from her brother. Sleep eluded her. On the rare occasions when she did sleep, imaginary men chased her in her dreams. No matter how creative she got with her hiding places, the dream invaders always captured her.

Soon April's body began to decompensate as well. She passed out often and shook a lot, almost as if she was having seizures. Specialists ordered lab work, neurologists ordered brain scans and EEGs, and a cardiologist, who diagnosed a heart murmur, hooked April up to a portable heart monitor she wore 24 hours a day. She was officially diagnosed with "reactive airway disease"—a variant of asthma—and prescribed half a dozen breathing medications meant to help with her light-headedness. But in spite of a variety of diagnostic tests and treatments, her symptoms persisted, baffling her doctors.

As April got older, she continued to live in a constant state of fear, immersing herself in seven different forms of martial arts, obsessed with becoming strong enough to protect herself. Fear convinced her to seek specialized protection training in a facility that focused on weapons instruction, evacuation scenarios, and hand-to-hand combat. She learned how to get into the minds of dangerous people, so she could protect others as a high-security bodyguard.

Every day, she strapped on a gun to go to work, willingly throwing herself in the line of fire on behalf of her clients. But even though April had become a highly skilled "executive protection agent," the fear didn't go away. If anything, she only grew more fearful, constantly looking over her shoulder, afraid to turn her back to anyone, certain that danger followed wherever she went.

She started sleeping with a gun by her bed, while nightmares of faceless men from the past still plagued her. She dreamed of being shot almost every night. She also developed a plethora of phobias—fear of the dark, of shadows, of spiders, of people standing behind her, of not being able to see people's hands. She started panicking whenever she had to leave the house, obsessively calculating and recalculating ways she might get attacked and how she might stay safe. She was terrified that if someone tried to hurt her again, she still wouldn't be able to stop them, in spite of all she had learned.

The more frightened April became, the sicker she got. Her fainting episodes worsened until doctors finally surmised that she was suffering from some strange blood disorder no hematologist had been able to diagnose. She wasn't bleeding, but somehow, her blood just disappeared, leaving her inexplicably anemic most of the time. To counteract whatever was going on in her body, doctors ordered infusion treatments, necessitating that she be hooked up to an IV machine three times a week in six-to-eight-week blocks for hours at a time.

April remembers looking out the window as a nurse tried for the third time to find a vein on her bruised, blown-out arm. The nurses were required to make six attempts at starting the IV before they could give up and page the specialized IV team. For six years April had been going through this ritual, and the more time passed, the more frequently she needed the infusions. The problem was getting worse, and nobody had any clue why.

In all that time, nobody once asked April about what might *really* be making her sick. Assuming that her poor health, her fear, and her past were unrelated, April never thought to mention the nightmares that left her shivering and sweating at night, the flashes of violent memories that left her shaking, or the surges of adrenaline she could feel coursing through her body whenever the fear showed up. She didn't understand that every time she felt that rush of adrenaline darting through her system, it had started as a thought or feeling in her mind that got translated into a series of physiologic responses throughout her body. April didn't know enough about the physiology of her body to understand that every time a fearful thought or anxious memory entered her mind, disease-inducing hormonal responses got triggered, and that this repetitive triggering took a terrible toll.

THE STRESS RESPONSE

The body comes equipped with a natural mechanism called the "stress response," also known as the "fight-or-flight" response. Although Walter Cannon at Harvard first described it, Hungarian endocrinologist Hans Selye later expanded upon it, describing the role of the hypothalamic-pituitary-adrenocortical (HPA) axis when the body is stressed, a response Selye termed the "general adaptation response," or GAS.[1] As Selye explains in his book *The Stress of Life,* he used the term "stress" to mean the biologic response of the body to any psychic demand, be it a negative emotion such as fear or anger or a positive change such as a new marriage or the birth of a baby.

When faced with a threat like the ones April faced when outrunning her abusers, the amygdala in the brain experiences the emotion of fear. The brain then communicates this emotion to the hypothalamus, which secretes corticotrophin-releasing factor (CRF) into the nervous system. CRF then stimulates the pituitary gland, causing it to secrete prolactin, growth hormone, and adrenocorticotropic hormone (ACTH), which signal the adrenal glands to release the stress hormone cortisol, aiding the body's ability to navigate a threat.

When the hypothalamus is activated, it also turns on the sympathetic nervous system, causing the adrenal glands to release epinephrine (also known as "adrenaline") and norepinephrine. These neurotransmitters are responsible for the jolt you feel in your body when you nearly miss crashing your car or someone jumps out of the shadows and startles you. They increase pulse and blood pressure, while also causing a variety of other metabolic changes all over the body. Your respiratory rate increases and your bronchi dilate, allowing more efficient oxygenation of the blood.

When the sympathetic nervous system is activated, your nerves fire more quickly so signals transmit more efficiently. Because warming the skin isn't a priority in the face of a threat, the skin cools and goose bumps form. Because the body needn't bother with digestion or reproduction in the midst of a life-threatening crisis, blood vessels traveling to the gastrointestinal and reproductive tracts constrict, shunting blood preferentially to the heart, large muscle groups, and brain, allowing your heart to pump harder, your thighs to run faster, and your brain to think more quickly. Your pupils dilate so you can better spot an attacker or find your escape route. Your metabolism speeds up and energy sources, such as fat stores, are broken down to release glucose into the bloodstream, giving you a burst of energy so you can fight or flee from the threat.

Stomach acid increases and digestive enzymes decrease. Cortisol suppresses your immune system in order to reduce the inflammatory response that would accompany any wounds an attack on your body might inflict. The body also stops all routine maintenance, shutting off its natural self-repair mechanisms—the ones that fight infection, prevent cancer, repair broken proteins, and generally fend off disease. Makes sense. After all, there's no point wasting the body's precious energy preventing disease or healing an illness that already affects you if you're about to die anyway because there's a gun to your head or a mountain lion is chasing you.

All of these physiological responses to fear are adaptive and protective when your life is really in danger. But here's the kicker. *You're not designed to be frightened often.* Period.

Epinephrine is toxic in large amounts, damaging the visceral organs, such as the heart, lungs, liver, and kidneys. The changes in stomach acid and digestive enzymes can cause esophageal contractions, diarrhea, or constipation. And when the stress response is triggered repetitively, sometimes the bronchi spasm instead of dilating—as in April's case—leading to wheezing, shortness of breath, and chest pain. In primitive humans, when real danger threatened the physical body, the fight-or-flight mechanism was protective, but most of the time, in modern society, it's just the opposite. Your body wasn't built to withstand the effects of chronic fear and stress. And yet, if you're like most people, your body is running on overdrive much of the time, fearing imagined threats, such as financial loss, the demise of a relationship, a threat to your stability, a perceived health threat, or a loved one's death—fears that most of the time never actually come true.

This leads to a vicious cycle. You fear getting sick, aging, or dying, and yet the fear can literally make you sick, age you, and kill you. Now, as you read this, you're probably even fearing fear itself! But don't worry. I'm going to help you understand how you can use fear to reduce stress responses and activate relaxation responses, so fear can help you grow, rather than making you sick.

THE NEUROSCIENCE OF CHRONIC FEAR

Neuroscientist Joseph LeDoux, whose book *The Emotional Brain* describes how the brain processes emotions, has studied the physiology of fear extensively. LeDoux describes the amygdala as "the hub in the brain's wheel of fear." All primal emotions, such as fear, hate, love, anger, and courage, arise from the amygdala in the limbic brain—the primitive, animal part of the brain. This fear hub works in conjunction with the thalamus, which receives information; the cerebral cortex, which reasons; and the hippocampus, which remembers.

Repetitive triggering of the stress response makes the amygdala even more reactive to apparent threats. Fear flips on the stress response, which triggers the amygdala—on and on and on. As this happens, the amygdala, which helps form "implicit memories"—fragments of past experiences that lie beneath our conscious recognition—becomes increasingly sensitized and tinges those memories with heightened residues of fear. As a result, fearful feelings, often manifesting as feelings of anxiety, exist even in the absence of any objectively fearful experience.

Simultaneously, the hippocampus, which is critical for developing "explicit memories"—clear, conscious recollections of what actually happened—gets worn down by the body's repetitive stress responses. Stress hormones like cortisol weaken neuronal synapses in the brain and inhibit formation of new ones. When the hippocampus is weakened in this way, it's much harder to produce new neurons, thereby making new memories. As a result, the chronic, painful, fearful experiences the sensitized amygdala records get programmed into implicit memory, while the weakened hippocampus fails to record new explicit memories.

When this happens, over time, you may wind up feeling chronically fearful and anxious, with no real memory of why you're even afraid. You may feel an overwhelmingly pervasive sense of doom and gloom, as if something bad—something *very bad*—is threatening you, even though, to an objective observer, you appear safe. Even long after the threat is over, anything that triggers this fearful response, consciously or unconsciously, stimulates the thalamus, which stimulates the amygdala and retrieves the fearful memory from the hippocampus, and suddenly—*BAM*. The body goes into hyperdrive. The trigger may not be directly related to the initial experience. It can be as simple as the feeling of a turtleneck around the neck or the scent of a fragrance that unconsciously stimulates the old memory. Once triggered, the physical reaction that follows is a warning system malfunction, alerting us to dangers that don't actually threaten us. This false fear is nothing more than a thought, but it leads to a potent stress response that affects not just your mind, but your body.

As a result of this warning system malfunction, false fears may take over the nervous system, contributing to phobias, post-traumatic stress reactions, anxiety disorders, depression, and other psychiatric conditions. No matter how much willpower you have and how motivated you are to heal, you can't just will yourself to be free of these kinds of fears, because the fear stems from unconscious processes and hooks into the most primal part of the nervous system. Even knowing that the fear is irrational doesn't help, because the fear response is bypassing the cognitive mind, going straight from zero to terrified in the primal nervous system, without engaging the thinking, rational forebrain. Something as seemingly harmless as a song playing on the radio can shunt the nervous system into past trauma and tinge even the most benign experience with the residue of fear, triggering stress responses. It's important to recognize that such responses are completely unconscious. If you're ruled by these kinds of fear reactions, you're not doing anything wrong. You're just stuck in a malfunction of your nervous system, and you'll likely need professional help in order to rewire it.

THE RELAXATION RESPONSE

Fortunately, the body has a natural antidote to stress responses triggered by fear, which Harvard professor Herbert Benson called "the relaxation response." The relaxation response counterbalances the fight-or-flight stress response, shutting off the sympathetic nervous system and switching over to the nervous system's relaxed state, the parasympathetic nervous system.

In its naturally relaxed state, the body is beautifully designed to repair itself. The body breaks down in small ways all the time. Cells go haywire. Toxins build up. Organs get damaged. We make cancer cells. We're exposed to pathogens and foreign bodies. Yet, the body knows how to handle such routine breakdowns. When the body is physiologically relaxed and not focused on outrunning a threat, our self-repair mechanisms kick in and naturally fend off illness. But as we've just seen, *the body's self-repair mechanisms stop functioning properly when fear remains unchecked. Only when the mind and body are relaxed can the body heal itself.*

When fear subsides and positive emotions replace negative ones, such as when the conscious forebrain experiences love, connection, intimacy, pleasure, faith, meaning, and hope, the hypothalamus stops triggering stress responses. Cortisol and epinephrine levels drop, the sympathetic nervous system shuts off, and the parasympathetic nervous system starts running the show. When this happens, pulse and blood pressure drop, blood is once again shunted back to less essential processes, such as digestion and reproduction, and the immune system flips back on. In this relaxed state, the heart is less stressed, the stomach produces less acid, and the body can go about the business of healing itself, returning to the homeostasis of optimal health.

In *Mind Over Medicine,* I shared the scientific data that proves how feeling states such as loneliness, work stress, pessimism, fear, depression, and anxiety can all trigger stress responses, while positive belief, loving connection, healthy sexuality, creative expression, gathering together in spiritual community, and meditation can initiate relaxation responses. When the mind shifts from fear to love, the mind can heal the body, and it's not some fuzzy New Age metaphysical thing. It's simple physiology.

While true fear is always protective and not something you want to lose, false fear can make the body sick if you don't know how to handle it in a healthy way. But if you learn to reframe your relationship to false fear, you can train your body to quickly abort the stress responses that accompany fear and shift to self-healing relaxation responses instead. When fear becomes the finger pointing at the issues in need of healing in your life, and when you're brave enough to let it transform you, fear has the potential to relax the nervous system as the mind focuses on healing solutions rather than scheming up more doom and gloom.

In Part Two of this book, you'll learn specific tools for transforming limiting beliefs into courage-enhancing truths in order to facilitate this shift from fear to love. In Part Three, you'll follow the Six Steps to Cultivating Courage to put these practices into action. As you do, you'll not only calm your mind and revive your spirit; you'll make your body ripe for miracles.

FEAR, ANXIETY, WORRY, AND STRESS

According to the Centers for Disease Control and Prevention, 80 percent of visits to the doctor are believed to be stress-related. Yet, as we discussed in the Introduction, what is "stress" if not fear, anxiety, and worry dressed up in more socially acceptable clothing?

Worry stems from our ability to turn something over in our minds in order to try to figure it out. This ability can be healthy when it's focused on problem solving without any fear-inducing thoughts accompanying it. But the minute problem solving starts inducing imaginary negative outcomes, it isn't just solving problems; it's creating them. Anxiety is an emotional feeling of nervousness, unease, dread, or apprehension. It's that sinking feeling we've all had that says, "Oh no. This could be *bad*." Stress can accompany worry or anxiety, but it refers to the physical response of the body as it responds to a real or perceived danger. Fear is defined as an unpleasant emotion that stems from a belief that someone or something is dangerous, likely to cause pain, or threatening to your safety, security, or happiness. Fear, anxiety, worry, and stress may have different dictionary definitions, but as far as the body is concerned, worry, anxiety, and fear all trigger the physical response of stress.

Fear rules our whole culture, so nobody is immune. We're afraid of unwanted pregnancy, date rape, and infertility. We're afraid of gay marriage, socialized medicine, and electing the wrong president. We fear failure, success, withering away into obscurity, and failing to discover our true purpose in life. We're afraid of financial disaster, but we're also afraid of making too much money. We're afraid to dream big, but we're terrified of not being extraordinary enough. We're afraid of expressing our creativity because we fear judgment or making mistakes, yet we fear keeping the song within us unsung. We're afraid of dying, but we're even more afraid of living.

You don't have to have a diagnosed mental illness to be afraid. Every human being naturally experiences fear as a survival mechanism. In some individuals, though, fear escalates into full-blown psychiatric conditions. Twenty-eight percent of Americans suffer from an anxiety disorder, which manifests when a person feels fear and experiences the physiological effects of it without any certain or immediate external threat of death or injury.[2] In addition to fearing things that could kill us, we're also afraid of public speaking, heights, going out in public, needles, and spiders. In fact, a 1986 study by the National Institute of Mental Health showed that 5 to 12 percent of people surveyed had experienced phobias in the past six months. There are as many as 530 documented phobias, and studies estimate that 24 million Americans will experience phobias in their lifetimes.

Women experience anxiety two to three times more frequently than men, but phobic disorders are equally common in men and women.[3] The ten most common phobias are arachnophobia (fear of spiders), ophidiophobia (fear of snakes), acrophobia (fear of heights), agoraphobia (fear of situations in which escape is difficult), cynophobia (fear of dogs), astraphobia (fear of thunder and lightning), trypanophobia (fear of injections), social phobias (fear of social situations), pteromerhanophobia (fear of flying), and mysophobia (fear of germs or dirt).[4] Some people even suffer from phobophobia, the fear of phobias![5] Other common anxiety disorders include generalized anxiety disorder, post-traumatic stress disorder, panic disorder, obsessive-compulsive disorder, and social anxiety disorder.

When fear leads to a full-blown psychiatric disorder, it's not just a finger pointing toward what needs healing; it's a bomb thrown into your life, interrupting your serenity and requiring you to call in the experts. Specific treatments for psychiatric conditions like these are beyond the scope of this book, but if you are suffering from the painful effects of such a disorder, or if someone you love is, please seek professional help. In addition to working with a therapist, there are many wonderful books written by experts that focus specifically on each of these psychiatric conditions. If you need it, I strongly encourage you to seek out this type of support, which you may then add to your Prescription for Courage as a part of how fear can cure you. The way I see it, we all have tools in our toolbox, and the more tools we add to our Prescription for Courage, the more likely we are to be successful in leading a life ruled not by fear, but by the soul's wisdom.

In the next chapter, I'll be sharing with you data proving that fear isn't just a painful emotion that causes psychological turmoil; it can be a serious risk factor for disease when not appropriately channeled. This information is not intended to scare you. It's meant to shift your perception so you realize that every fearful thought is triggering a stress response that puts your body in jeopardy, so you'll be motivated to let fear help you by writing and implementing your Prescription for Courage, rather than unconsciously being fear's victim.

Chapter 2 is meant to offer you a paradigm shift, one that illuminates the prevalence of fear in our lives and acknowledges that if we wish to live long, optimally healthy lives, addressing our fear is arguably more important than what we eat, whether we exercise, how many vitamins we take, or how many bad habits we have. I understand that it's radical to suggest that unchecked fear may lie at the root of many diseases. I'm not suggesting that these diseases don't also have biochemical roots, but I am suggesting that fear predisposes you to those harmful biochemical influences. Even more importantly, I'm suggesting that you can do something about this. You are not at fear's mercy. There's no need to feel helpless in the face of fear. Remember, fear has the potential to free you from suffering, and when you let it, your body will thank you.

CHAPTER 2

SCIENTIFIC PROOF FEAR CAN MAKE YOU SICK

The fact that the mind rules the body is, in spite of its neglect by biology and medicine, the most fundamental fact which we know about the process of life.

— FRANZ ALEXANDER, M.D.

In a case study described in the scientific literature, a subject described as "Baltimore Case Study Number 469861" was an African American woman born on Friday the 13th in the Okefenokee Swamp near the Georgia-Florida border. She was the third of three girls delivered that day by a midwife who proclaimed that all three, born on such a fateful day, were hexed. The first, the midwife announced, would die before her 16th birthday. The second would not survive her 21st. And the patient in question was told she would die before she turned 23.

The first two girls died within one day of their 16th and 21st birthdays, respectively. The third woman, terrified that she would die on her 23rd birthday, showed up at the hospital the day before her birthday, hyperventilating. Soon afterward, before she turned 23, she died, proving the midwife's predictions correct.[1]

Would she have died anyway from the heart and lung abnormalities found on autopsy? Or was she literally scared to death as a result of the hex put on her by the midwife? Was the whole thing one big nocebo effect (the opposite of the placebo effect— something meant to harm, rather than heal the body)? Was the midwife's hex akin to the voodoo deaths often reported in primitive cultures, when a witch doctor curses a villager, and the villager subsequently dies?

It's hard to say, but the three girls are certainly not the only ones to have reportedly died as the result of fear. The same thing happened to Mary Parnell, who had an unexpected encounter with 20-year-old Larry Whitfield. Whitfield had just been thwarted in his attempt to rob the Fort Financial Credit Union in Gastonia, North Carolina. Apparently, a bank staff member, seeing two men approaching armed with semiautomatic weapons, locked the security doors and alerted the cops, leaving Whitfield and his accomplice on the street holding loaded guns, with the cops on the way.

The two failed bank robbers jumped into their car and sped off down Interstate 85—until they made the rookie move of wrecking their getaway car and found themselves stranded. Whitfield, now on foot and looking for a place to hide, barged into the home of Mary Parnell, a 79-year-old grandmother of five, who was terrified by the intrusion of a stranger into her home.

"I don't want to hurt you," Whitfield reportedly said to Parnell, directing her into the bedroom and ordering her to sit in a chair. This may have been true, but all evidence appeared to the contrary in the eyes of Parnell. Wide-eyed and petrified, she promptly died of a heart attack. Her husband returned home four hours later to find her slumped over in the chair Whitfield had ordered her to sit in. Doctors listed her cause of death as "heart attack due to stress by home invasion."

Two lives are now over. Mary Parnell is dead, and Larry Whitfield has been sentenced to life in prison, convicted of scaring Mary Parnell to death.

SCARED TO DEATH

Can a person really be scared to death? Apparently, yes. Countless case studies in the medical literature report stories of frightened or terrorized individuals who died instantly. In a 1971 review in *Annals of Internal Medicine,* George Engel compiled the accounts of 170 case studies of deaths due to "disrupting life events," in categories ranging from acute grief to personal danger to the loss of status or self-esteem.

Some of the people studied by Engel died quite simply from fear. A 43-year-old man died after his 15-year-old son faked a kidnapping call, telling his father, "If you want to see your son alive, don't call the cops." A terrified three-year-old died in the dentist's chair while having baby teeth extracted. A four-year-old, afraid of the rain, died in a severe downpour.

A 63-year-old security guard was bound by robbers and died. A woman, seeing teenagers outside her apartment beating and robbing a bus driver, died while phoning the police. A 35-year-old man accused of robbery told his lawyer, "I'm scared to death!" Then he fell to the ground and died. A 45-year-old man, about to give a speech, apparently died of stage fright. A 72-year-old woman died after her purse was snatched.

Several survived brushes with death, only to die shortly afterward. Four men died right after automobile accidents in which they were not injured. A 71-year-old died after firefighters arrived at his house for what turned out to be a false alarm. An uninjured 55-year-old man, who walked out of an overturned railway car after a train wreck, died right beside the tracks.

Others in Engel's study died from acute shock and grief. A 14-year-old girl dropped dead when told of her 17-year-old brother's sudden, unexpected death. An 18-year-old girl died right after being told that her 80-year-old grandfather, who helped raise her, had passed. One of the owners of the motel in which Martin Luther King, Jr., was assassinated collapsed and died from a cerebral hemorrhage upon hearing the news. A healthy 39-year-old who had lost his twin the week before died suddenly himself. As he cradled the head of his son, who had just been injured in a motorcycle crash, a 40-year-old father slumped over dead.

Widely accepted as one of the experts in the phenomenon of sudden death occurring after life-altering events, Harvard professor Martin A. Samuels, M.D., has also been collecting stories from the lay press about people who may have been frightened or excited to death. Because his data is currently unpublished, I asked if he would share with me some of the stories he had uncovered so far. They include deaths on amusement park rides, deaths following brutal attacks, the death of a morgue worker after finding a live person on a slab in the morgue, and a death occurring during a showing of the movie *The Passion of the Christ*. Clearly, extreme emotion can be fatal, but how does this happen?

Experts claim that cardiac malfunction is usually the culprit, so let's explore the relationship between fear and the heart.

WHEN FEAR STRIKES AT THE HEART

Christopher was a 56-year-old resident of Chicago with a history of cardiac arrest that resulted from a potentially fatal arrhythmia. Lucky for Christopher, when his heart stopped functioning properly and he passed out, he was in a Michigan Avenue shopping mall that was equipped with an emergency defibrillator and someone trained to use it. When emergency medical personnel arrived, someone had already saved his life.

In the cardiac care unit of the hospital, Christopher's heart rhythm got out of whack again, prompting a Code Blue. An EKG showed that his heart was in ventricular fibrillation, which is when the ventricles quiver and shake, rather than pumping blood rhythmically as they should. Such a rhythm usually results in death, but Christopher was lucky. He was resuscitated, and as a way to try to prevent sudden cardiac death in the future, doctors implanted into Christopher's body a defibrillator capable of assessing his heart rhythm and, should it detect a lethal malfunction, delivering an electrical shock to stabilize the rhythm.

Christopher was released onto the streets of Chicago to go about life as usual with the hope that, should his heart malfunction, he'd get shocked, and while that shock might ruin his dinner date, it would save his life. Such was the state of Christopher's heart when he arrived at his office to see everyone hovering around the television, watching CNN as it played and replayed the collapse of the World Trade Center towers.

As the second tower fell, Christopher felt fearful, and his heart started palpitating. He dropped to the ground, just in case his defibrillator was about to go off, hoping he'd prevent himself from being injured from a shock-induced fall. But the shock didn't happen that morning. It finally came on September 14, when Christopher was at home, watching the news while lying on his sofa.

It was the first time Christopher's defibrillator had shocked him since he had been released from the hospital months earlier. Fortunately, it saved his life.

Was it pure coincidence that Christopher's heart started beating in a potentially fatal rhythm right after September 11 while watching the news? Researchers say no.

A study published in the *Journal of the American College of Cardiology* set out to determine whether the fear and anxiety the September 11 terrorist attacks left in their wake increased the frequency of sudden death in patients at risk of cardiac arrhythmias, specifically those patients fitted with implantable cardioverter defibrillators as a result of previous potentially lethal cardiac events. Researchers examined the patients' EKG readings before and after the trauma and found that, in the 30 days before September 11, 3.5 percent of them experienced ventricular arrhythmias. After September 11, 8 percent did—a 2.3-fold increase in risk.

These patients were New Yorkers, but it wasn't just those near the sites of the September 11 attacks who were affected. A similar study of people with implanted defibrillators in Florida also found an increase in ventricular arrhythmias remote from the scene of the disaster.

Twenty years earlier, another study shed similar light on what can happen when fear strikes at the heart. On January 18, 1991, after the United States launched Operation Desert Storm in the first Gulf War, Saddam Hussein ordered Iraqi troops to rain down 18 Scud missiles while the unsuspecting people of Israel slept. The terror of the missile attack came as a total surprise, and it was the first attack on Tel Aviv in Israeli history, representing a massive breach in national security.

Although there were no deaths directly related to the bombings, the people of Israel were terrified when the smoke cleared. Fear and anxiety ran high. Sales of Valium skyrocketed.

Interested in exploring the effects of fright on mortality rates, researchers at the Hadassah Medical Center in Israel tracked mortality rates in January and February of 1991, in the days following the surprise missile attack. Their findings, published in the *Journal of the American Medical Association,* showed that, unrelated to injuries sustained during the bombings, mortality rates increased by 58 percent—a 77 percent excess in women and a 41 percent excess in men—in the aftermath of the attack.[2] While the researchers posited that some of this increase could be explained by other factors—excessive physical activity as people ran from the missiles, missed medication doses, breathing difficulties induced by gas masks, and extended stays in sealed rooms without adequate oxygenation—they concluded that the primary explanation was fear's harmful effect on the body's physiology.[3]

Another Israeli study, published in *Lancet,* also examined the consequences of the Iraq strike on Israel and confirmed a sharp rise in the incidence of heart attacks and sudden death in the time following the attacks, when compared with five peaceful control periods.[4] Similarly, after two strong earthquakes shook Greece in 1978, a study published in the *International Journal of Epidemiology* showed a significant increase in mortality, not due to earthquake-related injury, but to deaths from "all other pathological causes," including heart disease.[5]

ANXIETY, PHOBIAS, PANIC DISORDER, AND HEART DISEASE

Ken grew up in a home where looking over your shoulder was a lifesaving mechanism. If he wasn't on constant alert, his father would sneak up behind him, usually after imbibing half a bottle of bourbon, and beat the crap out of Ken. Once Ken had been beaten to a pulp, he'd move on to Ken's younger sisters or his mother. As a child, Ken learned that it wasn't safe to sleep or to play or to ever let down his guard.

It's not surprising that Ken started experiencing panic attacks by the time he was a teenager. The attacks showed up with a sense of impending dread, followed by a gripping feeling in his chest; a racing heart; a nauseous feeling in his belly; a tightening of his throat; a cold, clammy, sweaty sensation; and a fearful feeling so potent he wanted to crawl out of his skin. These episodes happened without warning, and when they came, Ken felt certain he was about to die.

Fear of the attacks led him to avoid going out. His biggest fear was that he'd have an attack while trapped somewhere he couldn't escape. As a result, he avoided airplanes, subways, even freeways without frequent exits. The only place he felt safe was in his apartment, so increasingly, Ken just stayed home.

But even at home, the attacks paralyzed him. So he became increasingly anxious about having people over, fearful that they would witness him in the midst of a panic attack. Even though he was painfully lonely, he stopped inviting people over. By the time he turned 40, Ken had essentially locked himself in a prison of his own making, fueled by his fear of . . . pretty much everything.

This kind of phobic anxiety leads not only to emotional suffering; it may also lead to illness and premature death. While fear is natural, and everyone experiences moments of fear, some people like Ken feel fearful on a regular basis, and these frightened, anxious people have been well studied. Countless studies link anxiety, phobias, panic disorder, and heart disease. The U.S. Health Professionals Follow-up Study examined 33,999 men with high levels of phobic anxiety over a two-year period of time and found a two-and-a-half-fold higher risk of coronary heart disease, including a sixfold increase in sudden cardiac death.

Similar findings were demonstrated in the Normative Aging Study, which documented a threefold to sixfold increased risk for heart attack and sudden cardiac death among highly anxious patients.[6] The British Northwick Park Heart Study, published in the *British Medical Journal,* followed 1,457 men with phobic anxiety for six years. Among the most anxious men, this study found a 3.8 times higher risk of heart disease, particularly sudden death.[7] And after two years of studying approximately 40,000 men, researchers from the Harvard School of Public Health found the risk of sudden cardiac death to be six times higher in men who suffered from phobic anxiety. In a number of studied cases, victims died as a result of their phobias, with fatal heart attacks coming immediately after psychological stress. Most of them had no previous evidence of heart disease.[8]

Because much of the research on anxiety and heart disease had been done on men, another group of researchers at Harvard decided to prospectively evaluate 72,359 women from the famous Nurses' Health Study, all free of heart disease, over a period of 12 years. This study, published in *Circulation,* found that women with severe phobic anxiety showed a 52 percent increased risk of sudden cardiac death and a 30 percent increased risk of fatal coronary heart disease compared with less frightened women, confirming that it's not just men who can die from fear.[9] It doesn't help that those who suffer from heart disease tend to get anxious, and experiencing anxiety after a heart attack triples the overall mortality rate, doubles the rate of recurrent heart attack, and increases the risk of sudden cardiac death sixfold.[10]

The data is copious and clear. Fear and anxiety significantly increase the risk of heart disease and death.[11] But how does this happen? How does an emotion originating in the mind translate into heart disease in the body?

THE PHYSIOLOGY OF FEAR AND THE HEART

You already know how the stress response is initiated. You have a thought like *I'm afraid I'm going to lose my job* or *I'm afraid my child will die* or *I can't leave the house; it's too scary out there.* Suddenly, the gears of your wildly complex brain whir into action. The amygdala, the fear center of your brain, lights up. And boom—the stress response kicks in.

But how does the stress response translate to sudden death? Two competing theories have emerged to explain how people can be scared to death. In 1942, Walter Cannon, who first described the fight-or-flight response, published a paper entitled "'Voodoo' Death," in which he postulated that death by voodoo was caused "by a lasting and intense action of the sympathico-adrenal system."[12] In other words, the fear of being cursed to death stimulates the sympathetic nervous system into an extended stress response that literally wears out the heart.

In 1957, Carl Richter argued the opposite, based on work with rats. After being confined in glass swimming jars from which there was no escape, the rats often died suddenly. Electrocardiograms taken while the rats swam showed that their heart rates dropped, rather than raced, prior to death, and removing the adrenal glands didn't protect the rats. This was taken as evidence that overactivity of the sympathetic nervous system was not the cause of these deaths. Instead, Richter postulated that it was an increase in vagus nerve stimulation, ruled by the parasympathetic nervous system. When the vagus nerve is activated, everything drops—heart rate, blood pressure, respiratory rate, metabolic rate. When everything slows down too much, you black out, and in rare cases, you can even die.[13]

Who's right? Is the sympathetic nervous system the culprit? Or is it the parasympathetic nervous system?

It's not so cut-and-dried. We now know that the two are not mutually exclusive, and when the body senses a threat—even an imagined one—the whole nervous system goes haywire. Multiple studies suggest that most emotionally charged experiences initially cause stimulation of the sympathetic nervous system, triggering a stress response. But over time, when the stressor is prolonged as it was for the rats trapped in the swimming jars, the parasympathetic nervous system can take over, leading to dangerous slowing of the heart rate and respiratory rate and lowering of blood pressure. Both nervous system extremes can predispose to cardiac arrhythmias and sudden cardiac death.

There are other ways fear can strike at the heart as well. Patients with anxiety have been consistently shown to have excessive production of catecholamines, such as epinephrine and norepinephrine.[14] They also exhibit an exaggerated response to stress, with higher levels of stress hormones, which can tax the heart with elevations in heart rate and blood pressure.[15] What happens when the heart is flooded with too much epinephrine? Epinephrine binds to the receptors of cardiac myocytes (heart-muscle cells), causing calcium channels in the cell membranes to open. Calcium ions rushing into the cardiac myocytes cause the heart muscle to contract. If massive amounts of epinephrine bind to the heart cells, calcium keeps pouring into the cells, causing the heart muscle to stay contracted, leaving it unable to relax. When this happens, the nerve tissues on the heart—specifically the sinoatrial node, the atrioventricular node, and the Purkinje fibers—can start to wreak havoc on the heart, causing potentially lethal cardiac arrhythmias. Even with no history of heart disease, it's possible to just drop dead. It's also postulated that fear or anxiety may lead to sudden cardiac death by causing hyperventilation, which can induce coronary spasm and trigger a heart attack.[16]

It may sound complicated, but really it's quite simple. A thought originates in the mind, affects the nervous system, and damages the heart. It's just one of many potent, dangerous examples of the mind-body connection in action. And the heart is far from the only place where fear can strike.

DOES FEAR CAUSE CANCER?

Janet always feared cancer. Over the years, she performed all kinds of anti-cancer rituals—taking vitamin D supplements, wearing sunscreen, eating broccoli—almost as if bargaining with God while trying to keep fear at bay. But it wasn't just cancer she feared. After being pushed down a flight of stairs when she was a year old by her toddler brother, she had never felt safe in the world. She was afraid of illness, pain, anything that might cause cancer, anything toxic, unlocked doors and windows, intruders, and a host of other unnamed potential dangers. She feared doing things wrong and the shame and embarrassment that accompany imperfection. On her first-grade report card, her teacher had written, "Janet will one day find that it's a waste of time to worry so much about making a mistake."

Janet's fear manifested as chronic tension in her body, a sort of habitual clenching, particularly in her stomach and pelvic region, as if she could ward off fear and control her world that way. She once had the thought, *If I ever have health problems, they will stem from my stomach and pelvis.*

Sure enough, that was where she got sick. It started with a ruptured, necrotic appendix. Then one day, years after menopause, she started bleeding vaginally. Deep down, she knew the sleeping beast she had been tiptoeing around her whole life had finally awakened.

Just prior to her diagnosis of uterine cancer, she had gotten married to the love of her life. Although she was thrilled about getting married, her wedding generated great anxiety, as her perfectionist tendencies emerged, along with her fears that she might now lose the man she loved. The fear voice in her head had a constant mantra—*Be careful.*

Janet strongly suspected that fear had weakened her immune system and allowed her uterine cancer to take hold in her body, but that realization didn't stop the fear from getting worse. She had always feared doctors, needles, hospitals, and pain, and those things were now a regular part of her life. So it didn't surprise her when, a year after aggressive treatment, her cancer recurred. It made sense to Janet that when an area of the body is chronically tense, we block the flow of energy, oxygen, and circulation to that part of the body, leaving it vulnerable to illness.

Janet suspected that her cancer would win if she couldn't learn to deal with her fear. Because she already intuited that fear could be her friend, she turned FEAR into an acronym—"Feel Everything And Recover." Her cancer journey required her to fully face her worst fears, one breath at a time, one trembling foot in front of the other. She now finds that she is no longer clenched with fear; instead, she is embracing it, becoming fully present with it, and learning from it. And she is now cancer-free.

Janet believes fear caused her cancer, and her courage is helping her heal. But is there any data to support a link between fear, anxiety, and cancer?

This question sent me back to the medical journals, where I found a Norwegian study conducted through the University of Bergen. This study followed 62,591 people from one county of Norway who took part in a medical survey between 1995 and 1997, a survey originally used to develop the Norway National Cancer Registry, which listed participants who had developed cancers or premalignancies that might one day become cancers. Those involved in the study also underwent psychological testing to determine if they were anxious—and researchers found that the most anxious people surveyed were 25 percent more likely to have abnormal cells that might become cancer.[17]

There's less data specifically looking at fear and anxiety, but the medical literature is loaded with studies evaluating "stress" and cancer—and as we've already determined, the amygdala can't tell the difference between stress and fear. Whether it's work stress, stress from the loss of a loved one, the stress of a divorce, the stress of an empty nest, the stress of feeling lonely, financial stress, the stress of inadequate self-care, the stress of a health diagnosis, or the stress of being chased by a cave bear, the primal brain interprets it all as "THREAT!" And the stress response is triggered.

Because so many patients diagnosed with breast cancer are convinced that stress caused their cancer, researchers have studied this link in particular, looking for correlations between cancer and life stressors. A case-control study from Finland, published in *Psychotherapy and Psychosomatics,* examined the lives of 87 breast cancer patients and concluded that they had endured significantly more stressful life events, losses, and difficult life situations in the six years prior to the onset of disease than had population controls. The study found a survival advantage for those breast cancer patients whose lives were less stressful before diagnosis. The study was small, however, limiting the ability to make sweeping generalizations.[18]

A larger Polish case-control study, published in *Cancer Detection and Prevention,* interviewed 257 breast cancer patients who underwent surgery between 1993 and 1998 and compared them to 565 cancer-free controls. This study found that the breast cancer patients who experienced significantly stressful life events were 3.7 times more likely to develop breast cancer than those who didn't.[19]

An even larger study seems to confirm this correlation. Published in the *American Journal of Epidemiology,* it investigated the relationship between stressful life events and risk of breast cancer among 10,808 women from the Finnish Twin Cohort and found that those who experienced stressful life events in the 5 years before the initial assessment were more likely to develop breast cancer over the 15 years during which they were followed, especially if the stressors included the death of a spouse, close relative, or friend. There was also an association between breast cancer risk and divorce or marital separation.[20]

Not everyone in the scientific community is in agreement on whether stress predisposes people to cancer. Some data supports this hypothesis, while other data refutes it. Polly Newcomb, Ph.D., the head of the cancer prevention program at the Fred Hutchinson Cancer Research Center in Seattle, set out to definitively answer this question. Using trained interviewers to question women with cancer, as well as healthy women who served as controls, about the stress in their lives that preceded a cancer diagnosis, Newcomb asked nearly 1,000 study participants about stressful life events. Had they lost a loved one? Gotten married or divorced? Lost a job or retired? Gone bankrupt?

The results were clear. There was no association between self-reported stressful events in the previous five years and a diagnosis of breast cancer.[21]

But critics didn't buy it. They argued that Newcomb's study measured stressors, but not stress itself. Newcomb conceded that they had a point. She had made the understandable assumption that stressful life events equaled the physiological experience of stress—the fight-or-flight stress response. She'd used the assessment of stressful life events as a surrogate for what might have been happening in the body, but she hadn't actually measured what was happening in the body.

We might logically assume that if a person experiences a life stressor, this leads to more fear and more stress responses and might predispose him or her to cancer. But individuals deal with stress very differently. When you let fear become your teacher, allowing it to illuminate anything in need of healing in your life, stressful life events may even relax the nervous system because on some deep level, you know you're growing. Studies make it hard to control for this kind of adaptive response. Perhaps one person remains physiologically calm—with the body dominated by relaxation responses—in the face of a horrific life stressor, while another freaks out and gets flooded with stress responses as the result of an event others might deem stress-free.

After all, it's not easy to measure the physiological experience of stress when assessing stressors that happened before a patient enrolled in a study. Unless you enroll cancer-free patients in clinical trials ahead of time, hook them up to continuous monitoring, and follow them around over extended periods of time to see whether they develop cancer, it's hard to gather clean data that allows you to make blanket statements such as "Life stressors cause cancer." What we can conclude, however, is that the actual experience of stress can indeed put you at risk of disease, although perhaps the way you experience stressful life events determines your body's physiological response even more than the stressful life event itself. Perhaps if you let fear help you heal emotionally, mentally, and spiritually, stressful life events need not predispose you to health problems. Maybe, instead of leading to a breakdown, stressful life events can break you open, and your health can even improve. Such variables are difficult to test in research settings, which may explain why the data is mixed with regard to fear and cancer.

THE IMMUNE SYSTEM AND CANCER

Leonard's wife died in childbirth when she was only 42, leaving behind a 3-year-old, a newborn, and Leonard. On Tuesday, he was a happily married, expectant father, and on Wednesday, he was a widower and a single parent with a full-time job that left no room for grieving or parenting. In a panic, he hired a full-time, live-in nanny while trying to keep his head above water at work.

At first, his boss was compassionate, offering to give him time off to recover, telling him to do whatever he needed in order to heal from the shock. But once he came back to work, he felt the strain of expectation and knew he wasn't quite up to snuff. His numbers weren't as good as they usually were, he had trouble focusing, and there were younger, smarter, more qualified people in the corporation vying for his position. His instincts told him that his job was at risk, and as it turned out, his instincts were correct.

Six months after his wife had died, Leonard lost his job. Six months after that, he was diagnosed with lung cancer. Leonard is convinced that the stress of losing his wife, being left to raise his children alone, and losing his job and financial security contributed to his cancer diagnosis.

He's not the only cancer patient I met who feels this way. But do stress, fear, and anxiety actually *cause* cancer? In order to causatively link them, we need plausible biological mechanisms explaining how emotions like fear and anxiety might predispose someone to cancer. The mechanism most commonly postulated by scientists is immune system suppression resulting from stimulation of the stress response triggered by fear or anxiety. In the presence of such emotion, stimulation of the sympathetic nervous system negatively affects cancer-fighting lymphoid tissue and suppresses cancer-blasting natural killer cell activity.[22]

If you respond emotionally to a life stressor with fear and anxiety, the brain flips on the stress response, thereby weakening the immune system. When this happens, the body's tumor defense systems are weakened in turn. After all, every day, our bodies are exposed to carcinogens in the environment in which we live, and stray cancer cells develop regularly. When our immune systems are healthy, these rogue cancer cells are quickly and efficiently recognized and destroyed, long before a tumor develops, in one of three primary ways. Immune cells aim to prevent invading agents from entering the body in the first place. If cancer-causing agents do break through, abnormal cells can be repaired, or killer T cells can eliminate cancer cells.[23]

Seems simple, right? Fear and anxiety, left unexamined and unhealed, weaken the immune system and interfere with the body's ability to heal itself.

Or maybe not. Although scientists have long believed this explanation, newer data suggests it may not be so clear-cut. Copious evidence links stressful events with weakening of the immune system,[24] but the link between stress and cancer is actually quite controversial. The National Cancer Institute reports, "Although studies have shown that stress factors, such as death of a spouse, social isolation, and medical school examinations, alter the way the immune system functions, they have not provided scientific evidence of a direct cause-and-effect relationship between these immune system changes and the development of cancer."

A relationship between emotional stress and cancer is biologically plausible in principle. It's just that studies clearly demonstrating how stress might lead directly to cancer are lacking. There is substantial evidence that stressful life events are indeed associated with alterations in immune function.[25] But whether immune suppression actually predisposes to diseases is more controversial.[26]

That said, multiple studies do suggest immune mechanisms for how stress might predispose someone to cancer.[27] If a healthy immune system is required in order to fight off cancer, then it would stand to reason that people known to have suppressed immune systems would be at greater risk of cancer, and the evidence suggests that this is, in fact, the case.

Organ transplant patients taking immunosuppressive drugs to reduce the risk of organ rejection have intentionally suppressed immune systems. They also experience a greatly increased risk of cancer when compared to the general population. One Australian study, published in the *Journal of the American Society of Nephrology,* evaluated 481 kidney transplant recipients in the Australian Multicenter Trial of Cyclosporine Withdrawal who each received one of three different immunosuppressive treatment regimens. A total of 226 patients developed at least one cancer at rates much higher than the general population. By 20 years post-transplant, 27 percent of patients developed cancers that didn't include skin cancer, and 48 percent of patients developed skin cancer.[28]

Other data suggests that the lifetime incidence of a non-skin cancer after a kidney transplant ranges from 20 percent after 10 years to 30 percent after 20 years. That number rises to 65 percent if you include skin cancers. Even if someone survives their kidney failure and dangerous transplant surgery, cancer is the cause of death in 70 percent of transplant recipients who are diagnosed with a non-skin cancer, and among those who survive, the battle with cancer can be difficult in the face of a weakened immune system.

Compared with non-transplant recipients, kidney transplant patients have a 15-fold increased risk of Kaposi's sarcoma, lymphoma, skin cancer, and kidney cancer, while melanoma, leukemia, hepatobiliary, and female genital tract cancers are five times more likely. Common cancers that affect the general population—such as those affecting the gastrointestinal tract, prostate, pancreas, and breast cancer—are also increased, though to a lesser degree.[29]

Other immunosuppressed patients, such as those with AIDS, also experience higher rates of cancer, mostly the types of cancers known to be related to infection, such as stomach cancer, associated with the bacteria Helicobacter pylori; liver cancer, associated with infection with the hepatitis B and hepatitis C viruses; Kaposi's sarcoma, associated with herpesvirus 8 infections; lymphoma, associated with Epstein-Barr virus; and cervical cancer, associated with human papillomavirus.

Such data strongly suggests that a healthy, functioning immune system is necessary to fight back cancer. But other data muddies the waters.

If emotional stress causes cancer by suppressing immune response, it would be reasonable to assume that people who had
experienced stressful life events, such as losing a child or having
a child with a serious illness, would be at higher risk. With that
in mind, researchers studied such people. One Denmark study
published in the *New England Journal of Medicine* examined the
incidence of cancer in 11,380 parents whose children had cancer.
Certainly, researchers posited, the parents were guaranteed to experience physiological stress, and this should show up as a higher
risk of cancer. But parents in this study were no more likely to
develop cancer than the general population.[30]

A second Danish study published in the journal *Cancer* evaluated cancer rates among 21,062 parents who had lost children.
Following these parents for up to 18 years afterward, researchers
found a slight increase in cancer risk in mothers, but not among
fathers who had experienced such a tragedy.[31]

So we can't definitely say that stress, fear, or anxiety causes
cancer—but there *is* evidence that they can help it progress.
A study in the *Journal of Clinical Investigation* shows that stress
hormones known to be associated with such emotions, such as
epinephrine, can directly support tumor growth and spread.
For normal cells to thrive in the body, they need to be attached
to neighboring cells. Cells that detach from their environment
undergo a form of programmed cell death. But cancer cells can
bypass this programmed cell death, allowing them to break off
from cancerous tumors and float around the body, through the
blood or lymph system, spreading to distant sites, leading to cancer metastasis.

Studying cells exposed to stress hormones, Anil Sood, M.D.,
from the University of Texas MD Anderson Cancer Center, found
that such cells were also protected from programmed cell death
and could survive unanchored to neighboring cells. Sood hypothesized that this would increase the chance of tumor spread. To test
this, he and his team transplanted ovarian cancer cells into mice,
who were then restrained in order to subject them to fear and
anxiety. In response, their tumors grew more quickly than tumors
in mice not subjected to such emotional stress.[32]

So, does stress cause cancer—or does it make cancer more likely to spread? The data doesn't permit us to make as clear a causal link between fear and cancer as we can between fear and heart disease. But one thing is incontrovertible. Unless you learn to let fear be your teacher, fear may weaken your immune system and increase your cancer risk. But if fear can help you break through to the truth of who you are, it may be just what the doctor ordered.

STRESS AND RESPIRATORY INFECTIONS

Other links between fear and disease are easier to draw. We know that emotional stress weakens the immune system, so it makes sense that infectious diseases normally fought off by a healthy immune system occur more commonly when you're stressed out. We've all been there. You're anxious about your work or you're afraid your father is going to die from the heart attack he just had or you're worried about your marriage, and then, THWACK! You get a cold or a sinus infection or pneumonia.

In an Australian study published in *Psychosomatic Medicine,* 235 adults aged 14–57 years affiliated with three suburban family physicians in Adelaide, South Australia were identified as either high stress or low stress, based on a questionnaire, then followed over six months to see who got sick. Not surprisingly, the high stress group experienced almost twice as many sick episodes (2.71 vs. 1.56) and almost twice as many days of symptoms (29.43 vs. 15.42) as the low-stress group.[33]

To determine whether stress predisposes people to the common cold, researchers at Carnegie Mellon reported in the *New England Journal of Medicine* their findings after studying 420 healthy people who were assessed for their degree of stress, including their exposure to past stressful life events, as well as their current emotional states, including such emotions as "scared," "nervous," "angry," and "distressed." They exposed 394 of the study participants to one of five cold viruses, while 26 were exposed to a placebo. Researchers evaluated who got sick and who didn't; those who were stressed were more than twice as likely to get sick as those who weren't.[34]

STRESS AND CHRONIC DISEASE

The average American experiences 50 stress response episodes each day, and because the body's natural self-healing mechanisms are deactivated during a stress response, this can take its toll on the body over time. Frequent elevations in blood pressure result in thickening and tearing of blood vessel walls, which can lead to organ damage. Cortisol causes excessive production of fatty acids and glucose, which can predispose you to elevated blood sugars, putting you at risk of diabetes and its complications, such as blindness and kidney failure. Through the effects of high levels of cortisol, chronic stress responses can make it very difficult to maintain a healthy weight, putting you at risk of obesity, which increases the likelihood of many other health conditions. Chronic stress responses can also lead to muscle tension and inflammation, causing a variety of chronic pain conditions and musculoskeletal disorders.[35] Chronic stress responses can also increase the risk of thyroid disease, ulcers, autoimmune disease, sexual dysfunction, depression, anorexia nervosa, Cushing's syndrome, and inflammatory diseases.[36]

Repetitive stress responses even affect the aging process. In a Harvard study examining the data of 121,700 nurses from the Nurses' Health Study, patients were assessed for the presence of phobic anxiety in forms such as panic disorder and agoraphobia. Researchers from Brigham and Women's Hospital analyzed survey results and blood samples from 5,243 women, ages 42 to 69, and found that intense phobic anxiety leads to faster biological aging, as measured by the marker of leukocyte telomere length, DNA-protein complexes on the ends of chromosomes believed to be biological markers of aging.[37]

Although some diseases have not been well studied, it's likely that chronic stress responses exacerbate *all* chronic diseases, even the ones that may have clear biochemical explanations, such as genetic disorders. In order to optimize health, the body needs to be in relaxation response the majority of the time so the body's natural disease-fighting mechanisms can operate properly.

STRESS AND OTHER SYMPTOMS

It's not just heart disease, cancer, and chronic illnesses that are impacted by emotional stress. When exposed to stress, the body tends to whisper before it yells. Stress often manifests through less immediately life-threatening physical symptoms, such as backache, headache, eye strain, insomnia, fatigue, dizziness, appetite disturbances, and gastrointestinal distress. Consider the following physical symptoms, which are all potential side effects of chronic repetitive stress responses—whispers from the body signaling the potential for more serious diseases in the making.

TEN SIGNS YOU HAVE WAY TOO MANY STRESS HORMONES

1. You're not sleeping well.

Cortisol levels are supposed to drop at night, allowing your body to relax and recharge. But if your cortisol levels are too high, you might notice that, even if you've been tired all day, you get a second wind right around bedtime. Then you toss and turn all night—and feel tired again the next day. Scientists theorize that higher levels of ACTH and cortisol triggered by the stress response also reduce surges of nighttime melatonin levels and thus encourage insomnia.

2. Even when you sleep well, you're still tired.

Not only can stress cause insomnia, which leads to fatigue; over time, high levels of cortisol deplete the adrenal glands and may result in "adrenal fatigue syndrome," a condition related to stress that is rarely acknowledged by conventional medicine. Chronic stress can lead to feelings of exhaustion, even in the face of adequate sleep time.

3. You're gaining weight, especially around your abdomen, even when you eat well and exercise.

Cortisol tends to make you thick around the middle, even when you're doing everything "right." Cortisol raises your blood sugar, putting you at risk of diabetes. High glucose

---

levels then bump up your insulin levels, which in turn drop your blood sugar, and all of a sudden—yes, you guessed it—you're struck with wild cravings for Twinkies. Stimulation of the sympathetic nervous system may also cause the stomach to release the amino acid ghrelin, which makes you feel hungry and can lead to weight gain, especially if you tend to numb negative emotions with food.[38]

4. You catch colds and other infections easily.

Cortisol deactivates your body's natural self-repair mechanisms, which means that that immune system perfectly designed by nature to keep you healthy goes kaput, leaving you vulnerable to every pathogen you encounter.

5. You feel dizzy for no good reason.

Stress can manifest as occasional dizziness or even chronic vertigo, most likely as a response to changes in the autonomic nervous system stimulated during stress responses.[39] Alterations in vital signs, particularly elevations in respiratory rate, can lead to hyperventilation, which can alter the acid/base balance of the body and affect the nervous system's responses to balance and coordination via the cerebellum and the eighth cranial nerve.[40]

6. You experience backaches and/or headaches.

When your cortisol levels are high over a long period of time, your adrenal glands start to get depleted. This raises prolactin levels, increasing the body's sensitivity to pain, such as backaches and muscle aches. Excessive cortisol also hypersensitizes the brain to pain, such that even the slightest twinge can excite the nerves of the brain, causing headaches.

7. Your sex drive disappears.

Consider cortisol the anti-Viagra. When stress hormones are high, libido-inducing hormones like testosterone drop, and voilà . . . nothing.

8. Your gut acts up.

Your gastrointestinal system is very sensitive to stress hormones like cortisol. Stress commonly leads to gastrointestinal distress in the form of nausea, heartburn, abdominal cramps, and diarrhea. The effect on the gastrointestinal system is most likely mediated by the increased amounts of ACTH generated during the stress response: in response to ACTH, the stomach empties less effectively, leading to stomachaches and abdominal cramping. Heartburn can occur not only because stomach acid levels increase, but also because activation of the sympathetic nervous system reduces the stomach's pain threshold, increasing the perception of pain in response to heartburn and predisposing you to stomach ulcers.[41] The stress response also restricts the stomach's ability to expand, which in turn stimulates contractions of muscles in the colon that can lead to diarrhea and bowel cramping.

9. You feel anxious.
Cortisol and epinephrine can lead to jitters, nervous stomach, and feelings of panic, even paranoia.

10. You feel blue.
High levels of cortisol suppress production of serotonin, and next thing you know, your mood takes the plunge into feelings of sadness. Over time, this can even predispose you to clinical depression.

In accordance with what I believe about how fear can help you, there's evidence that how we feel and think about stress has a lot to do with how it affects us physiologically. In a 2013 TED talk, health psychologist Kelly McGonigal shared that according to one study, people who experienced a lot of stressful life events in the previous year had a 43 percent increased risk of dying— but this was only the case for people who *believed* that stress was harmful for their health. In fact, people who experienced many stressors but did not view stress as harmful were no more likely to die than those who had relatively few stressful circumstances in their lives. In fact, the stressed-out people who weren't worried about their stress had the lowest risk of dying of anyone in the study![42] In other words, it's not life's stressors per se that make us sick and miserable. It's the stories we make up about these events, which translate into negative beliefs that activate chronic repetitive stress responses, shorten our life expectancy, and lead us into despair.

Researchers extrapolated this data and estimated that over the eight years they were tracking deaths, 182,000 Americans died prematurely, not from stress itself, but from the belief that stress is bad for you. If that estimate is correct, then the belief that stress is bad for you accounts for more than 20,000 deaths per year, making it the 15th largest cause of death in the United States in 2013. That's how powerfully belief affects the body. In other words, it's our thoughts and beliefs, not the fear-inducing life stressors themselves, that make us sick. In light of this data, framing fear as something that can wake you up and help you grow may even offer a survival advantage. We'll talk more about this crucial aspect of The Fear Cure in Part Three.

FEAR AND HEALTH CARE

Not only can unfettered fear cause illness; fear can also lead patients to seek out too much medical care, and it can cause doctors to dole out too much treatment. In *Overdiagnosed: Making People Sick in the Pursuit of Health,* doctors H. Gilbert Welch, Lisa M. Schwartz, and Steven Woloshin compare such vigilant pursuit of diagnosis to the warning lights on modern-day cars. Because automotive technology has advanced so far since the days when you could tinker with your car in your own garage, these sophisticated sensors can identify automotive abnormalities long before the car's performance is affected. The warning lights are, in essence, making early diagnoses.

Sometimes, this can prevent a major breakdown. By diagnosing a problem early, you can avoid getting stranded on the side of the road, waiting for AAA. And as one who hates nothing more than getting stuck on the roadside, I appreciate the times those little lights have helped me avert disaster.

But, according to my auto mechanic, early diagnosis is not always a good thing. Several times when the warning lights on my own car have gone on, he has examined it and deemed the alerts "overdiagnoses." Because my mechanic is ethical, he didn't charge me anything in those cases or replace a part that didn't need to be replaced. He did warn me that if I wanted to be absolutely 1,000 percent safe, I could put my car through a procedure that might prevent future problems. But in his estimation, the car might go another two or three years before whatever triggered the warning light became a real and present danger—if it ever did.

We face similar choices in health care. As the authors of *Overdiagnosed* say, "If we doctors look at you hard enough, chances are we'll find out that one of your check-engine lights is on." The harder you look, especially when it comes to cancer screening, the higher the likelihood that you'll wind up diagnosed with something that may or may not cause problems in the future.

Once upon a time, people only sought medical attention when they had symptoms. Routine physicals and screening tests are a relatively new phenomenon. The quest for early diagnosis and preventive intervention all started with high blood pressure: once doctors discovered a link between high blood pressure, heart disease, and stroke, measures began to be taken to screen asymptomatic individuals and convert them into patients. And without question, such measures have been lifesaving. For those with severe high blood pressure, even if they are asymptomatic, the likelihood of experiencing an adverse event is dangerously high. Treatment can prevent early death.

But diagnoses such as hypertension are based on numbers. In years past, high blood pressure was only treated if it was severe—systolic blood pressures greater than 160 or diastolic blood pressures greater than 100—or if there was evidence of "end organ damage," such as eye, kidney, or heart problems. Then, in 1997, the Joint National Committee on High Blood Pressure took a hard stand, strongly admonishing physicians to treat even individuals with mild hypertension—those with blood pressures just over 140/90, without evidence of end organ damage. That one change meant that an additional 13 million Americans suddenly qualified for anti-hypertensive treatment.[43]

Who decides which number makes you normal and which makes you abnormal? Here's where things get a bit arbitrary—and potentially dangerous. Because doctors have hammers, and everything tends to look like a nail, there's a tendency to keep lowering the cutoffs for numbers-based diagnoses like hypertension, diabetes, hypercholesterolemia, and osteoporosis. As a result, the number of asymptomatic individuals labeled with these diagnoses—and treated for them—is rising, without substantially reducing the number of deaths these conditions cause. To many patients, early diagnosis and early intervention, designed to prevent long-term adverse events, feels protective, safe, nurturing even. But more diagnosis means more treatment, which means more complications from treatment, which means more iatrogenic health conditions, those caused by the very medical treatment meant to help them.

Entering the health care system as a patient is not an entirely benign procedure under any circumstances, given the risk of medical error. Nobody likes to talk about it, but if medical error were listed as a separate cause of death, it would rank as the third most common cause of death in the U.S., just behind heart disease and cancer. In 2010, the Office of Inspector General for Health and Human Services reported that up to 180,000 deaths annually are attributable to medical error.[44] The Institute of Medicine's widely quoted 1999 report "To Err Is Human" was more conservative in its estimate, reporting that up to 98,000 people die each year as a result of hospital mistakes (which would make it number six among top causes of death).[45] Most recently, in 2013, the *Journal of Patient Safety* reported that 210,000–400,000 premature deaths result from preventable medical error.[46] It's possible that these numbers would be even higher if we included the often unreported consequences of what happens outside of hospital settings. Very simply put, the fear that makes us want to aggressively protect our health can make us sicker.

Fear plays a particularly big role when we're talking about cancer, which research has shown to be the most feared disease in

America.[47] "Carcinophobia"—fear of cancer—is a relatively new phenomenon, and it has led to remarkable strides in medicine, fueling research that has led to a cure for some cancers. Yet the advances in cancer diagnosis and treatment are shadowed with a dark side—overdiagnosis and overtreatment.

A study published in the *Journal of the National Cancer Institute* estimates that 25 percent of breast cancers detected on mammogram, 50 percent of lung cancers diagnosed by chest X-ray and sputum analysis, and 60 percent of prostate cancers diagnosed by prostate-specific antigen (PSA) are "overdiagnosed." The authors of the study define "overdiagnosis" as "the diagnosis of a 'cancer' that would otherwise not go on to cause symptoms or death." It is not the same as misdiagnosis, which implies that the pathologist made a mistake looking at the specimen under a microscope. Overdiagnosis suggests that the cancer exists, but that it is clinically irrelevant—that left untreated, either it would regress spontaneously (we know this happens) or the patient would die of something else before the cancer caused harm. All too often, these overdiagnosed conditions are treated with medically unnecessary procedures that reduce patients' quality of life, including radical surgery and treatments such as chemotherapy and radiation that are known to predispose to other cancers in the future. The authors of the study conclude, "Whereas early detection may well help some, it undoubtedly hurts others."[48]

Early studies back in the 1980s suggested that screening mammography reduced breast cancer mortality by up to 25 percent. More recently, the U.S. Preventive Services Task Force estimated the reduction at about 15 percent.[49] But those figures were based on outdated assumptions about the progression of the disease. In fact, the authors of *Overdiagnosed* report, for every 2,000 women invited to screen for breast cancer over a period of ten years, one death from breast cancer will be avoided—but 10 healthy women, who never would have become symptomatic or died from their disease, will wind up diagnosed and treated for breast cancer unnecessarily.[50]

A Norwegian study that compared 109,784 women who were screened only once in six years to another group of 119,472 women who were screened every two years found that the group that got more mammograms had 22 percent more invasive breast cancer diagnoses than the group that got screened only once. How do you explain this? The Norwegian researchers concluded that the more frequent mammograms found some invasive breast cancers that would have disappeared if left untreated. In other words, as shocking as this seems, some invasive breast cancers would have spontaneously resolved if they hadn't been detected first.[51] Responding to the concern for overdiagnosis and overtreatment, the U.S. Preventive Services Task Force changed its recommendations in November 2009. The new guidelines no longer recommend screening low-risk women younger than 50 or older than 75, and among women 50–74 years of age, mammograms are recommended not yearly, but every other year. They also recommend against teaching breast self-examination to patients.[52]

The data for prostate cancer is even more disturbing. Prostate cancer is so common that many men never even know they have it. In one study, pathologists in Detroit examined the prostates of 525 men who had died not from prostate cancer, but from accidents. None of these men had been diagnosed with prostate cancer while they were alive, but of those in their 20s, almost 10 percent had prostate cancer when pathologists went looking for it. Of the subjects who were in their 70s, over 80 percent had prostate cancer.[53] If this many older men have prostate cancer but only 3 percent of men will ever die from prostate cancer, something doesn't quite add up.

As with early diagnosis of breast cancer, early diagnosis of prostate cancer with PSA (prostate-specific antigen) did not change the rates of late stage cancer deaths. Instead, since 1975, when PSA screening began, an additional two million men have been diagnosed with prostate cancer.[54] In *Overdiagnosed,* H. Gilbert Welch concludes this: "My best guess, given the data, is that for every man who benefits from screening by avoiding a prostate cancer death, somewhere between thirty and a hundred are harmed by overdiagnosis and treated needlessly. That does not strike me as a good gamble." In an article in *The New York Times* entitled "The Great Prostate Mistake," Richard Albin, who discovered PSA testing, takes a similar line, writing, "The test is hardly more effective than a coin toss. As I've been trying to make clear for many years now, PSA testing can't detect prostate cancer and, more important, it can't distinguish between the two types of prostate cancer—the one that will kill you and the one that won't."[55] Fortunately, the medical establishment finally realized the great prostate mistake. In May 2012, the U.S. Preventive Services Task Force finally recommended against routine PSA screening in asymptomatic men.

When you examine the data, you can't help wondering whether we're so afraid of missing potential dangers to our health that our fear is causing us to do too much to protect it. Yes, it's wonderful that we have all the technology that we have. Every single doctor I know has many stories of how a screening test caught a potentially lethal disease early and perhaps saved a life. If that one patient is you or your loved one, it makes all screening tests seem worth it. But unless we're able to objectively examine the risks, benefits, and potential outcomes of such screening tests, our fear may cause us to deliver and receive bad medicine, in spite of all our best intentions to heal and protect.

Many patients are so afraid of getting sick and dying that if a doctor gives them the chance to screen for a potentially fatal illness—or even a health condition that might predispose to a lethal illness, such as high blood pressure, diabetes, or high cholesterol—they jump at the chance. More medicine is considered good medicine. The majority of doctors feel the same way. As doctors, we are motivated by the desire to be healing forces in the world. Our intentions are pure, but we're so afraid of making mistakes that we sometimes let fear drive us to order too many tests, prescribe too many drugs, perform too many procedures, and intervene when we might be better off taking a "wait and see" approach. And we simply don't know when to give up or even when to let someone die, rather than resuscitating over and over and over.

For both doctors and patients, our fear of death drives all of this. We are not okay with death, especially early or unexpected death. We consider death something to fight, not something to accept, and this potent fear fuels our entire health care system. This is a relatively recent phenomenon. Historically, doctors had access to much less technology, which meant that most diseases could be treated only with tonics, hope, and the love of someone who sat at the bedside and wiped a feverish brow. Now, in the age of technology, we're driven to keep treating, even when 90-year-olds with terminal conditions are hooked up to life support. In a real sense, untempered fear is not only harming our health from the inside, but from the outside as well.

THE GOOD NEWS

Now take a deep breath . . .

Don't let this data scare you. Let it be your wake-up call instead. You don't need to feel helpless when you feel afraid, because you can do something to let fear help you grow and heal. It's important to understand that fear in its many forms may be as much a risk factor for our health as smoking, eating Twinkies, or failing to exercise, but it's also critical to realize that fear is not something to avoid; it's something to lean into. As a culture, we need to develop a whole new relationship with fear, one that allows us to use fear as an opportunity for awakening, so we can come into right relationship with uncertainty, make peace with impermanence, and let the nervous system relax—even in the face of adversity. When we do this, the body can use its capacity for self-repair to the fullest. Part Two of this book will help you take the first step toward changing your relationship with fear so you can let fear wake you up rather than rule you. We'll start with some straight talk about the nature of fear—how to discern which fears protect us, where fear comes from, and how we can use it to advance our spiritual development. We'll then dive into four cultural beliefs that form the basis for most of our fears and investigate ways to transform these beliefs into the raw material for courage. By the end of Part Two, I hope you'll find yourself looking at the world through new eyes, in a way that helps you use fear as signposts along your path, steering you straight to your true purpose.

PART TWO

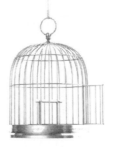

The **TRUTH**
ABOUT FEAR

CHAPTER 3

DISCERNING FEAR

If only we'd learned how to harness and ride rather than hunt and kill the butterflies that live in the gut of every person who strives to create something extraordinary from nothing.

— JONATHAN FIELDS

In June 2013, I was on my book tour for *Mind Over Medicine*, driving in a borrowed minivan from Chicago to an event in Indiana, where I was scheduled to speak to 300 cancer patients. I was tooling along on the freeway at 65 miles per hour, listening to music, feeling happy and calm, grateful for the opportunity to do work I love, enjoying the present moment. If I had been able to monitor my nervous system, I suspect it would have registered a relaxation response, with my parasympathetic nervous system dominating and my natural self-healing mechanisms doing their thing.

Then, in a split second, from out of nowhere, some unidentified piece of metal tore off another car and came flying right at the minivan. The unexpected road debris punctured both tires on the left side of the vehicle, causing it to list to the left, as if it might flip over.

Fear flooded through me, and I felt the rush of electric warmth as my fight-or-flight responses were triggered. If I had been hooked up to monitors, surely researchers would have been able to measure high levels of cortisol, epinephrine, and norepinephrine, and they would have noted that my heart and respiratory rate increased, my pupils dilated, my blood glucose levels spiked, and blood got shunted to my large muscle groups, giving me strength and fueling my ability to quickly maneuver the disabled minivan off the crowded freeway, where my life really was at risk.

A surge of energy and focused attention helped me grip the wheel and bring the car safely to the shoulder of the highway without getting hit or hitting somebody else. My body was out of danger at that point, so in an ideal world, researchers monitoring me would have noticed that, after 90 seconds, my stress hormone levels would start to drop, my vital signs would stabilize, and my nervous system would return to homeostasis with the parasympathetic nervous system in charge.

But alas, that isn't what happened. As I sat there, trembling from the rush of epinephrine coursing through my body, my imagination went nuts and my mind began to generate all the things that might go wrong now.

Here's a replay of what went on in my mind:

> *I'm going to miss my lecture and everyone's going to be upset at me. I'll disappoint the event planner and all those cancer patients who will be waiting for me to appear on stage. The friend I borrowed the car from is going to be angry with me for puncturing her tires and leaving her car stranded. Everyone is going to think I'm untrustworthy and unreliable. I don't even know who to call, since my purse was stolen in Miami and with it, my AAA card. I'm going to wind up stranded on this highway all night, in the freezing cold with no heat and no gas. I might even get attacked by some crazy person taking advantage of me in my vulnerable state. Plus, nobody is ever going to ask me to speak at an event like this again.*

The first wave of fear that rushed through me was what I've defined as "true fear" because it's the kind of fear that demands action and can help save your life. When the car was out of control and I was trying to get it safely off the road, my life really was in danger, and my stress response was appropriate. But the secondary fears that came up once I was safe were all what I call "false fear." These fears were just stories I made up in my mind, stemming from imaginary concerns that might or might not come to pass. Were these imaginary fears helpful? Were they going to help me avoid negative outcomes? No. There was nothing I could do to change the fact that I was stranded on the side of the road with 300 people anticipating my arrival in an auditorium 50 miles away. While the true fear that fueled my safe exit from the highway protected me, the false fear thoughts only kept me stuck in stress response. When you're in that state, it's nearly impossible to creatively problem solve. You're too busy trying to outrun danger to anticipate potential challenges in the future and calmly brainstorm solutions. And we've already seen how repetitive stress responses can harm your health in any number of ways.

Because false fear spirals like the one I experienced often happen unconsciously, I wasn't even aware at first of how one true fear that saved my life had resulted in a situation that triggered a dozen false fears. Once I realized what was happening, I took a moment to practice a brief relaxation response meditation so I could calm down my nervous system and allow it to reboot. This practice took me a few extra moments, which meant I was that much closer to missing my speaking appearance. But calming my nervous system was essential if I was going to critically assess the situation and focus my imagination on coming up with creative solutions, rather than dreaming up imaginary negative outcomes.

From this relaxed state, I was able to track down the AAA phone number and call a tow truck. I also realized I could call my friend and the event coordinator to see if either of them were available to help me out. My friend called her husband and he got in the car to meet me in Indiana, so he could oversee the car repair while I focused on getting to my speech. Once I had made my phone calls, it took another hour for the tow truck to arrive—more time to chill out and meditate, since there was nothing else I could do to hasten the process. If I kept breathing and focusing on the present moment, I could fend off false fear. But the minute I started thinking about the future, I got scared again. Because I knew I had already done everything within my power to get to my talk on time, I kept having to remind myself to calm down. I felt less afraid when I was able to stay mindfully in the moment and surrender control of the situation to something larger than me.

Finally, the tow truck arrived. The driver was a sweet, burly guy who smiled at me with kind eyes when I prattled on about what had just happened. "Climb in, darlin'," he said.

After dropping the disabled car off at the garage where my friend's husband was waiting, he said, "Don't you have a speech to get to?" Smiling, he told me his shift was over and offered to drive a half hour out of his way to take me to the performing arts center. I felt a rush of relief.

On the way to my event, the guy I nicknamed "Tow Truck Angel" asked what I was going to talk about, and I told him I was giving a lecture to cancer patients about how to optimize your chance for cure. Tow Truck Angel got teary and started telling me about his father, his best friend, whom he'd seen every single day until he died five years earlier of metastatic cancer. Tow Truck Angel showed me a clipboard adorned with photos of the Ford Mustang he and his father had built together before he died. He said, "I loved my dad so much."

He delivered me right to the door of the performing arts center, just in time for me to run my fingers through my roadside hair and walk up on stage fully relaxed. Not one of my false fears came true. I wound up telling my story to the audience, and the story of how I got there helped me demonstrate the very point I was trying to make with my talk: that the stress response triggered when my life was in danger was protective, while all the stress responses triggered by my false fears only caused unnecessary suffering in the moment and put me at risk of potential illness down the road. But those were also the fears pointing me toward things I needed to heal.

TRUE FEAR AND FALSE FEAR

True fear is a survival mechanism meant to protect you. It's the kind of fear an animal experiences when a predator stalks it, triggering the fight-or-flight response that may save its life. True fear is what you experience when your minivan goes out of control on the interstate. False fear, on the other hand, shows up as worry, anxiety, and ruminations about all the things that could go wrong in an imaginary future. It's always the finger pointing toward something that needs to be healed in your mind. In this way, both true fear and false fear can help you, if you know how to interpret them in healthy ways.

If someone could wave a magic wand and make you fearless, you probably wouldn't survive very long. Those who grow up to be diagnosed with antisocial personality disorder are often fearless as children, and such fearlessness puts them at great risk. Fear is critical to our safety and survival. But the very thing that protects you can go haywire. Although false fear can illuminate areas in your life that need your attention, healthy decisions that guide appropriate behavior never arise from false fear; they arise from intuition and integrity. Learning to discern between true fear and false fear allows you to know which voices in your head you can trust to guide your decisions.

True fear is the fear you feel as you lean over a cliff and realize that one misstep could kill you. It's the fear you feel when you meet a mountain lion on your hike. It's the fear you feel when someone holds a gun to your head. It can also be the calm, measured voice in your head that says, *This guy is dangerous* or *I need to go check on the baby right this second*. The voice of true fear is meant to keep you safe.

You may think that false fear keeps you safe too. Perhaps you think that worrying about your finances will keep you financially secure. Maybe you think that fear of having your child abducted leads you to take better care of him or her. You might think fear of getting sick keeps you from engaging in reckless behaviors. Maybe you think you're more likely to quit smoking or eat organic because you're afraid your health will suffer. Many people think fear is the only thing keeping them from reckless behavior that might threaten their career, their financial stability, their marriage, their quest for excellence, their reputation, their health, and the safety of those they love.

But does false fear really help you behave more responsibly? If you weren't afraid, would you throw away your money, leave your child unattended, and gorge on sugar? Is false fear what motivates you to make good decisions? And are the stress responses such fears activate worth the risk they cause to your body? No!

By shining a light on what needs to be healed, false fear may indeed play a role in helping you look at your money issues, your bad habits, your parenting challenges, and any dissatisfaction in a relationship. False fear may also alert you when creative problem solving is called for. If you can recognize it as a signal not to let stress responses run amok but to explore the situation further, in a calm, relaxed, intuitive way, false fear may have something to teach you. For example, maybe you're afraid about getting cancer, even though you just got a clean bill of health from your doctor. Perhaps the fear stems from an intuitive knowing signaling you that your unhealthy lifestyle may be putting you at risk of cancer, even though you don't have it yet. Maybe your instincts are telling you to stop eating so many processed foods, ditch the cigarettes, and start meditating so your immune system is better able to maintain healthy homeostasis. Or maybe you're afraid of running out of money, even though there's plenty of money currently in your bank account. Perhaps this is an alert from your intuition that the reckless way you've been spending needs to stop so you can build up more of a buffer in case something unexpected happens to your income stream.

The key is understanding that you don't need the fear in order to motivate healthy, responsible behavior, although it's worth paying attention to the fear that may point a finger in the direction you need to be looking. When false fear is in charge, your mind gets smaller. You limit your ability to problem-solve creatively. You're paralyzed into inaction. But when you're able to let fear help you expand your consciousness, something opens up, and you're able to make better decisions.

THE VOICE OF TRUE FEAR

While false fear can be useful for shining a light on areas of your life in need of healing, it's not false fear that motivates responsible decision making. It's integrity and intuition. These are what fuel you to take good care of your children, excel at work, commit yourself to healthy relationships, make sound financial decisions, and take care of your body. The voice that your intuition speaks with is the voice of the part of you I call your Inner Pilot Light. When you're tapped into this inner guidance system, it will steer you to make decisions that are aligned with your truth, and the good news is that fear can point you toward your Inner Pilot Light, if you learn how to bridge the two.

For example, let's say you find someone's wallet in the grocery store. Your fear of financial lack might make you think you should pocket the wallet, but if you learn to examine your fears consciously, you'll see that such fears point toward your growth edges. You may realize that your money fears are tempting you to compromise your integrity, but the more attuned you are to the voice of your Inner Pilot Light, the more likely you are to turn the wallet over to store security in case its owner comes looking for it. On the other hand, if you're out of touch with your Inner Pilot Light and your fear of financial lack is running the show, you might rationalize why you should keep the wallet and pocket the money. When you're tuned in to your Inner Pilot Light, this inner guidance system will help you do the right thing.

Keep in mind that the "right thing" might not correspond to society's rules. Your Inner Pilot Light enforces your soul's values, not those of society. The law might say that you shouldn't give money to beggars, but your soul might say you should. Society might say you should stay married until death do you part, but your Inner Pilot Light might steer you otherwise. How can you tell whether you're being guided by your Inner Pilot Light? Because it will feel good. Not in a short-lived, hedonistic, ego-gratification way, but as deep, nourishing soul-food fulfillment. You'll be able to tell the difference because following the voice of your Inner Pilot Light leaves you respecting yourself as well as others. Because your Inner Pilot Light can be trusted to protect you, this wise part of you will lead you to take any necessary precautions that will ensure the safety of you and your loved ones, and the good news is that this kind of guidance improves your health, rather than threatening it.

But while your Inner Pilot Light can be trusted to guide you, you'll have to learn to distinguish this voice from another, often much louder voice in your head, the voice of your Small Self. You could call this part of you your Gremlin, your Inner Lizard, your ego, or the voice of fear itself. I prefer calling it your Small Self because like a child, it *is* small and can't be trusted to make healthy, discerning, adult decisions. This is the voice that speaks loudest when fear is running the show, and it keeps you from taking in the useful messages your fear has for you.

YOUR SMALL SELF

Your Small Self doesn't need your judgment. It needs you to be your bigger self by acknowledging and tending it, rather than rejecting it or dismissing it. Your Small Self tends to be very frightened and is often reacting unconsciously to things that happened in your childhood. But your Small Self also develops in reaction to societal influences, adult traumas, and all of the ways we try to protect our self-image, our limiting beliefs, our relationships, our security, and our worldview. Any unhealed traumas from your past trigger false fears in the present, and your Small Self wants to ensure that you do a good job protecting what it values. This part of you tends to be irrational and psychologically immature. As a result, it chatters away 24/7, filling your mind with false fear thoughts, not because it's bad, but simply because it's a childish, hurt, scared, overprotective part of your psyche. As your Small Self adopts all sorts of additional "reasons" to be afraid in its quest to feel safe, you get a full-spectrum barrage of false fear erupting from this voice.

Your Small Self has the ability to imagine all sorts of possible disasters, and it thinks it's protecting you by warning you about all the impending awful things you should anticipate so your Small Self doesn't get hurt again. You don't even have to wait until problems arise before your Small Self starts giving you advice. It's already anticipating everything that *could* go wrong before anything bad even happens.

For example, even though I grew up in a happy home environment with two very loving parents, my Small Self grew up seeking approval and feeling like she was never quite good enough, no matter how much she achieved. My parents often reassured me that they loved me regardless of my achievement, but in spite of their reassurances, my Small Self kept trying harder . . . and harder . . . and harder, earning straight A's and being the good girl, going to medical school and graduating at the top of the class, and then becoming a successful author. And yet, for years, it was still never enough. I kept trying harder to win the approval not just of my loved ones, but even of strangers. Although I became aware of and was able to abort this unhealthy pattern in my professional life, it kept on running my personal life. I was trying harder and harder to win the approval of the men in my life, but no matter how much I sacrificed myself to demonstrate my devotion, I wasn't feeling loved enough in return. It wasn't the fault of the men. They were doing everything they could to love me. But none of them could heal my childhood wound.

With the help of my therapist, I was able to trace that pain back to my earliest childhood. I discovered that my Small Self was running the show in many of my relationships with men because false fear was driving her. When I tried hard to please a man and didn't feel appreciated, I would let my Small Self take the wheel and dictate my behavior in ways that my boyfriends perceived as irrational. They were right. My reactions were out of proportion to what was happening in present time because my Small Self was reacting not just to the present, but to old, deep hurt, and as a result, unnecessary stress responses were triggered. Once I was aware of how fear was sabotaging my relationships, I was able to use the realization fear granted me in order to break old patterns. I realized that, when my Small Self felt insecure in a relationship, my childhood fear of rejection led me to cling and grasp, which only pushed healthy people away. Once I recognized the pattern and where it came from, I was able to heal these childhood wounds. My goal now is to let my Inner Pilot Light call the shots in my relationships instead. In this way, my fear was a blessing. It was a billboard announcing to me how I was creating my own suffering and how I might shift those unhealthy patterns. While I still struggle with my Small Self, I'm on my way to healthier relationships, so I experience fewer stress responses in my relationship life, and I'm able to make more courageous decisions.

Unless you've done loads of therapy (and maybe even then), your Small Self probably still takes the wheel and dictates your behavior when he or she gets scared. Your Small Self tends to have its favorite scripts, and it repeats them *over* and *over* and *over* again. It's always worried about abandonment and rejection, because most of us never felt quite secure in the love of our parents, no matter how great Mom and Dad were. It's always worried about money, even if there's plenty of money in the bank, because most of us have unhealed childhood issues around financial security; even if we grew up wealthy, we were probably taught that we had to guard against financial loss. Your Small Self likes to tell you that you shouldn't make yourself vulnerable, because if you trust people, they could break your heart. Your Small Self is insecure, self-conscious, and self-absorbed, always trying to enforce the fear-based rules you learned in childhood. Your Small Self should not be automatically trusted to give you wise counsel, yet many people let this voice rule their lives without even questioning it.

While these are all opportunities to let fear point to areas that need healing in your life, the tricky part is recognizing when your Small Self takes the wheel and acknowledging that it can't be trusted to make good decisions. If you're letting your Small Self guide your behavior, you've turned over your power to an unreliable advisor—and to make matters worse, your Small Self is unaware of its limitations. It thinks it can handle making all your important decisions, and just to make sure you're paying attention, it talks to you *all the time.* To make things even more confusing, this voice likes to take two sides of an argument, so it will steer you first one way, then the other. Your Small Self is constantly playing devil's advocate to try to ensure safety and certainty.

In *The Untethered Soul,* Michael Singer writes, "You said to your mind, 'I want everyone to like me. I don't want anyone to speak badly of me. I want everything I say and do to be acceptable and pleasing to everyone. I don't want anyone to hurt me. I don't want anything to happen that I don't like. And I want everything to happen that I do like.' Then you said, 'Now mind, figure out how to make every one of these things a reality, even if you have to think about it day and night.' And of course your mind said, 'I'm on the job. I will work on it constantly.'" It's your Small Self that has given your mind this assignment. What results is a nonstop litany of false fear.

Because you're not aware that your Small Self is talking, its advice may sound rational, smart, protective, and worthy of implementing when you hear it inside your own mind. But what if someone wrote down the transcript of what your Small Self was saying? You'd probably find that what you're hearing sounds something like this:

> *This job sucks. I should quit. My boss doesn't respect me and keeps stealing my ideas. I deserve a promotion, but Bob got promoted instead of me. Bob is a schmuck who just kisses ass to get ahead. But wow. It worked for Bob. Maybe you should suck up to get ahead too. No, that would make me as much a schmuck as Bob is. I don't want to be a schmuck. I should just quit my job. But you can't quit your job. How would you pay the bills, you idiot? Plus, you'd be crazy to quit your job in this economy. Don't you know how lucky you are to have a job at all when unemployment is this high? You'd be better off sucking up like Bob and trying to get ahead so you don't have to work with that asshole boss who doesn't respect you. But Bob is a douche bag. Do I have to become a douche bag to get some respect around here? I really want to be a musician instead. What if I could play my guitar all the time and get paid for it? Now you're really talking crazy. Nobody gets paid to play the guitar. You think you're Carlos Santana all of a sudden? You should be grateful you have a good, stable job and*

a decent paycheck so you can feed the kids. But I hate my job. I should quit . . .

Underneath the chatter, though, your Small Self is really saying something much simpler—and if you listen, you can hear the fear clearly.

Things were always changing when I was young and unable to protect myself. I felt hurt and scared and insecure, so I want you to promise you'll keep me safe. I don't trust you when you think about changing things. My security feels threatened, and this frightens me. If you quit your job, I won't feel safe, so please don't change anything, even if you're unhappy. Listen to me instead and do what I say.

Once you realize what your Small Self is really saying, you can ask yourself what needs to be healed in order to move beyond these false fears. Perhaps you need to heal your tendency to grasp at security so you can find peace amidst change. Whatever it is, your Inner Pilot Light will guide your awareness so you can find peace beyond fear.

As another example of how your Small Self may operate, consider how you may be letting it prattle on about your relationships. Imagine the dictation of your thoughts on this topic.

Mark doesn't love me. If he loved me, he'd know how much I wanted to go to the movies tonight. But he didn't ask me to go to the movies. He went out with his friends instead. He loves his guy friends more than he loves me. If he loved me, he'd want to go to the movies with me. Maybe I'm not pretty enough. Maybe if I were prettier, he'd choose me tonight. I should color my hair. Maybe I'd be prettier if I was a blonde. But then I'd have those ugly roots. I hate it when fake blondes have dark roots. Mark would definitely not love me if I had dark roots. I shouldn't dye my hair blonde. I should work out more and lose weight. Then Mark will take me to the movies because I'll look more like Alicia if I work out and lose weight. Mark probably likes Alicia more than me. I'll bet he's wishing he could take her to the movies tonight instead of being with his friends. I'll bet he'll swing by Alicia's place after they're done.

Maybe they're having an affair. No, Mark wouldn't do that to me. He loves me. But if he loved me, he would have taken me to the movies. Maybe he really is having an affair. Maybe he's not even with his friends right now. I should call him. No, then you're just being a paranoid girlfriend nagging him when he's out with his friends. You should play it cool. Act like you don't really want to go to the movies. You should call Allen. Allen would take you to the movies in a heartbeat. But I don't love Allen. Yeah, but then Mark might think twice about choosing his friends over you. But I love Mark, not Allen. But Allen's really into you. Wouldn't it be nice to get some attention tonight? You should call Allen.

What your Small Self is really saying may be something more like this:

Dad was always criticizing how I looked, and it made me feel unlovable. Whenever anyone looks at another woman, I feel unloved and unlovable. Dad was always going out with his guy friends instead of paying attention to me. Whenever Mark goes out with his friends, I feel rejected.

What needs to be healed here? If you're not sure, don't worry. Your Inner Pilot Light knows, and we're going to be talking more about how you can learn to hear, interpret, and trust this voice.

Keep in mind that ignoring the voice of the Small Self doesn't help. Pretending you don't hear it only makes it scream louder. And while it's one thing to learn from the fears your Small Self is always obsessing about, it's a whole other thing to let those fears control you. You can see why it makes no sense to act on the immature, irrational advice of this hurt young voice.

If you've been taking orders from your Small Self, letting your false fears dictate your actions, don't beat yourself up. You can't help it if you've been letting your Small Self guide you. You didn't know any better. But now you do—and you can choose to change the voice you trust to give you advice. It's not too late to replace this immature advisor with a trustworthy mature one. Your Inner Pilot Light is always standing by, ready to take over as the best guide and counselor you've ever had.

COURAGE-CULTIVATING EXERCISE #1

Let Your Inner Pilot Light Nurture Your Small Self

1. When you recognize that your Small Self feels scared and is at risk of acting out, take a time-out. If you're in the company of other people, excuse yourself for a moment if you can, even if you have to find a restroom to have privacy. Cry if you need to. Let your Small Self feel angry or disappointed or betrayed. Then visualize the radiance of your Inner Pilot Light comforting your Small Self like a loving grandmother, a guardian angel, or the arms of Mother Earth holding your Small Self in her arms. Let her ask your Small Self what is needed—sleep, comfort, reassurance, permission to have a tantrum, a feeling of safety. Let your Inner Pilot Light tend to it, not in an indulging way, but the way you would comfort a hurt child.

2. Invite your Inner Pilot Light to see if there's anything the Small Self and its fears can teach you about what might need loving attention in your life.

3. Make a mental note of any messages your Inner Pilot Light has to share with you regarding your Small Self's fears. Put what you uncover on the back burner to be addressed later; in the moment, give priority to making sure your Small Self feels safe and comforted. Once your Small Self calms down, it's easier for your Inner Pilot Light to take charge and return to the situation as a mature adult, able to make brave decisions and behave courageously.

DRESS REHEARSING TRAGEDY

Human beings are the only species capable of imagining the future, which is both a blessing and a curse. Our ability to imagine and try to predict the future allows us to plan, reason, fantasize, and attempt to create stable lives for ourselves and our families. Imagination is the birthplace of creativity and problem solving.

Imagination allows us to turn problems over in our minds and consider creative solutions. Everything ever created by human beings began as imagination. This marvelous human ability has yielded genius inventions that make our lives easier, such as the wheel, the airplane, and the Internet. It has also birthed scientific advancement, solutions for seemingly impossible dilemmas, and timeless works of art, music, and culture. Even though we are arguably much weaker than other species from a pure strength perspective, we are rarely prey for other species anymore because imagination has allowed us to overcome our inherent vulnerability. Imagination also allows us to learn from past error, experiment with improvements, and avoid future problems. It helps us fend off unnecessary risks to our bodies so we can stay as healthy as possible. It helps us protect our children from harm.

But the very same imagination that has helped us evolve as a species torments us in a way that is unique to humankind. Consider how the imagination causes you to suffer unnecessarily in your love life. You fall in love, and the minute you realize how much you've given your heart to another human being, you recognize how vulnerable you are, and your Small Self starts acting up.

When I interviewed Anita, she started talking about the fears that pop up whenever she falls in love. She had been in a relationship with someone she really cared about for over a year, but she noticed how her Small Self was starting to sabotage her love life.

> *I love him so much I can hardly stand how risky this feels. What if I screw up and he stops loving me and leaves me? What if someone else more attractive than me steals him away? What if he discovers who I really am and sees what a basket case I am? I better keep my guard up. I better not tell him that one thing or he might leave. What if he gets sick? What if he dies? THIS IS TOO RISKY! I CAN'T HANDLE IT IF I LOSE HIM. I should just love him less. I should be prepared for when he leaves me, because I'm sure he will. I shouldn't let myself feel this much. I better keep my guard up. That way, if I get hurt, I'll be prepared.*

Brené Brown calls this "dress rehearsing tragedy." It's as if we hope that, by imagining the worst-case scenario, we will somehow prepare ourselves in case the worst does happen. Sometimes this actually can be an effective fear-reducing strategy, since at times, the looming undefined false fear of an uncertain future can be more terrifying than the specificity of the worst-case scenario. For example, when I was trying to decide whether to quit my job as a doctor, I was afraid of how I would pay the bills for my family. But when I really let myself dress rehearse the worst-case scenario, I realized that the worst thing that could happen was that I would wind up unemployed, bankrupt, and broke, and my family would have to move in with my mother. While this wasn't an appealing thought, it actually gave me courage because I realized the worst-case scenario wasn't really so bad.

I never did wind up living with my mother, though I did wind up $200,000 in debt before things turned around for me financially. Knowing that I could move in with my mother if the worst happened made me less frightened and enabled me to take the leap and quit my job. In such cases, dress rehearsing tragedy may ameliorate false fear.

But dress rehearsing tragedy has a grave shadow. In *Daring Greatly,* Brené Brown shares the following story written by a man in his 60s:

"I used to think the best way to go through life was to expect the worst. That way, if it happened, you were prepared, and if it didn't happen, you were pleasantly surprised. Then I was in a car accident and my wife was killed. Needless to say, expecting the worst didn't prepare me at all. And worse, I still grieve for all of those wonderful moments we shared and that I didn't fully enjoy. My commitment to her is to fully enjoy every moment now. I just wish she was here, now that I know how to do that."

WHOSE FEAR IS IT?

Where did the frightened voice of your Small Self come from? Why is this voice always spouting off false fears? It's enforcing a series of rules you learned in childhood, ostensibly to keep you "safe." Yet the false fears of your Small Self may not even belong to you. They may come from much farther back.

We tend to inherit fear like a virus that gets passed from generation to generation. We unconsciously take on the fears of our parents, often by the age of six, when their "programs" get downloaded into our subconscious minds without our consent. Such patterns can become the operating instructions for your entire life. Common operating instructions passed on from generation to generation include beliefs such as:

- Bad things happen when you're not in control.
- You'll be judged if you let yourself be vulnerable, so keep your guard up.
- Fly under the radar and don't ever rock the boat or all hell will break loose.
- Prioritize what's certain, secure, safe, and right, even if it makes you unhappy.
- You have to work your ass off in order to survive.
- Life doesn't work if it's pleasurable.
- Don't follow your dreams, because it's not realistic or responsible.
- Everyone is out to get you, so protect your heart at all costs.
- Self-sacrifice is good. Self-care is selfish.
- Don't enjoy sex or you'll go to hell.
- Be perfect or you might get rejected.

You may have inherited these fear-based rules from your parents, they inherited them from theirs, and unless you wake up, you'll pass your fears along to your own children, usually in the name of keeping them "safe."

These generational fears can show up as a result of a cultural trauma, such as the Holocaust. Many who have survived such genocides have passed on a fear of persecution, long after the real threat that once triggered true fear in the ancestors is gone. Financial lack represents another common generational fear. For example, those who survived the Great Depression had true fear about starvation and poverty, and they passed on a fear of lack to generations of plenty. This fear may show up as an insatiable need for more and more money, even when there's a bounty of food on the table and plenty in the bank.

Scientific evidence backs up this idea of generational fear. In a study conducted by Brian Dias and Kerry Ressler at Emory University, published in *Nature Neuroscience,* mouse parents were exposed to electrical shocks whenever they smelled the scent of cherry blossom and almond. Subsequently, the children and grandchildren of the scared mice startled in response to the scent of cherry blossoms, even though they had never been exposed to the scent or shocked when they smelled it. Offspring of the scared mouse parents also had more neurons that detected the cherry blossom scent than mice whose parents hadn't been shocked when exposed to that scent. Such fear can be transmitted at the level of the DNA: Researchers found that the DNA in the sperm cells was imprinted with the association between fear and the scent of cherry blossom. A gene that codes for the molecule that detects this odor carried a chemical marker that they postulated may have changed the behavior of the gene.[1]

The ability to inherit fear from your parents may have developed as a survival instinct, a way to learn what can threaten your life without having to be exposed to the threat, but in modern society, this biological adaptation has a dark side that may explain how seemingly irrational phobias, anxiety, and post-traumatic stress disorder develop—to say nothing of your everyday fears, such as fear of never having enough money or fear of being rejected by those you love.

However, as Bruce Lipton teaches in *The Biology of Belief,* you are not a victim of your genes. Just because your genes may have been programmed by your ancestors doesn't mean you're destined to abide by their rules. Even if your genes reflect the influence of these fears, how your genes express themselves depends on a variety of epigenetic ("above the genes") forces, which include your thoughts, beliefs, and feelings, your physical environment, and the people you surround yourself with. And once you realize that these fears don't even belong to you, you can start to let go of the past and focus on what's happening in present time. By letting fear illuminate what's in need of healing, not just in you, but in your family, you have the potential to heal not only yourself; you can break the chain of generational fear and heal your entire bloodline.

Becoming aware of the fears you've inherited from your ancestors isn't about blaming your ancestors or playing the victim. Your ancestors need your compassion, not your judgment, and you can be grateful that the fears you've inherited are helping you heal. Like you, your ancestors inherited these fears from their own predecessors. Awareness allows you to forgive them while reprogramming your subconscious mind, so you are free to act from a new set of operating instructions—the instructions of your Inner Pilot Light.

It's important to be gentle with your Small Self as it tries to impose its inherited rules and false fears. This part of your psyche needs your compassion too. Rejection only makes your Small Self act up. Instead, offer love. What will unfold is healthy decision making that takes into consideration appropriate precaution without letting false fear run the show. Part Three of this book will offer you tools for changing the unconscious operating instructions that may be guiding your life, healing from generational fear, and learning to trust your Inner Pilot Light. You'll learn further practical exercises that help you soothe your Small Self so you can discern appropriate action from a place of trust, rather than false fear.

WHAT DOES YOUR FEAR HAVE TO TEACH YOU?

When I first met Dennis Couwenberg at the Institute of Noetic Sciences holiday party, we were introduced several times. Since I was a physician author and he was the owner of an academic scientific publishing company, people suspected we would have a lot in common. They were right. We connected over our shared interest in the intersection of science and spirituality and our curiosity about various forms of anomalous healing, such as energy healing, shamanism, and whatever was happening at John of God. Dennis was recovering from a painful divorce, and his search for relief from the suffering of heartbreak thrust him onto the spiritual path through yoga and meditation. I was several years into my own spiritual journey and also in the middle of a divorce, so we became fast friends. Our initial meetings focused on intellectual matters. We shared with each other books that left our very skeptical scientific cognitive minds baffled and curious, and we'd spend hours hashing over things most scientists dare not touch, like the scientific data on telepathy, reincarnation, and near-death experiences.

Within three weeks of our first meeting, Dennis and I, alongside my friend April, had a spontaneous mystical experience that left all three of us confused, disoriented, ecstatic, and awed. Everything turned topsy-turvy in our lives, and as the fireworks subsided, Dennis and I found ourselves in a strange sort of spiritual partnership, where the purpose of our friendship became clear. We were here to illuminate all of the fears, childhood patterns, and limiting beliefs of the Small Selves that had been unconsciously operating our lives and creating our suffering. I was in the middle of writing this book, and Dennis became one of my willing case studies, demonstrating to me with brave commitment how fear can wake you up if you're willing to go into the dark places, shine light on them, and use what you find there.

At one point, Dennis had been happy in his job in scientific publishing, but as he grew to better know his own soul's essence, Dennis realized his business wasn't aligned with his true nature. This realization scared him. It's not easy to shift gears mid-career. He was familiar with publishing. He was well connected within the industry. He felt stable and secure in his ability to generate enough revenue to get by within his area of expertise. He dreamed of starting over, but fear kept getting in the way. What would he do if he stopped publishing scientific books? How would he pay the bills?

Dennis wound up taking a sabbatical from his work in order to get some perspective and gain clarity. He was fortunate to be self-employed, with money in the bank to fund a sabbatical, but after six months away from his business, he was watching his savings account dwindle. He was clear that he didn't want to return to his old job, but he had no idea how he would pay the bills when the money ran out. When Dennis spoke to me about his fears, I asked him to share what the voice in his head was telling him about the option of a career change. Here's what Dennis's Small Self was saying:

Who do you think you are? You think you have what it takes to really follow your dreams? You already took six months off and nothing good came of it. You've spent enough time acting out. It's time to come back to earth, cut your losses, and act responsible. Continue what you have been building up so nicely and know how to create money with, even though you don't like it too much now. This is the only way you know how to make money. There's no way out. This is how the world works. But what about the other people who follow their dreams, do what they love and get paid for it? I see other people who do this. This time I'm really passionate about doing something else. I want to love my job passionately. I feel really motivated to make it work this time. But doing what I love can't possibly make me money, Life just does not work like that. It might work for other people, but I'm not like those people. Life doesn't work for me when it's pleasurable. If I try to pursue my dream, I'll wind up broke and nobody will respect me. I will never get out of just scraping by, even if I try really, really hard. But I'm educated. Look how far I've come already. I've been in a marriage where things were really good, with plenty of money. My ex followed a passion in the artistic world and made plenty of money. I should be able to do this too. But I'm not like my ex. My ex has a different mind-set than me, as well as a supportive family. I'm not optimistic like that, and I don't have that family safety net. I don't believe in myself that way. My possibilities are very limited. A complete career change would never work. I will run out of money before any of my dreams come true. But I was the first person in my family to get an education. I started a publishing company that is unusually successful. But that's not special. Anyone could have done that. That doesn't mean anything. I will never make it if I try to follow my dream. I don't have enough drive. I feel energetically drained before I even get started. I don't know where to start. Unless I go back to my job, I'm going to wind up bankrupt and on the street. Then nobody will love me or respect me, and I'll never recover. At least if I stay in my publishing job, I'll be safe, even if I'm not that happy for now.

What was Dennis's fear trying to teach him? To discern this, first we looked at whether there was any validity to what Dennis's Small Self feared. He was not in any imminent danger. There was no tiger chasing after him. Nobody was holding a gun to his head. He still had food to eat, a warm place to sleep, and a substantial chunk of change sitting in his bank account. However, while he was safe in the present moment, he had never invested in buying a house, he didn't have any money in a retirement account, and unless he took some action in order to shore up his dwindling savings account, it was possible that Dennis could run out of money.

Sure, an unexpected business opportunity or an inheritance from a relative he didn't know he had could show up on his doorstep with no planning on his part. When my friend SARK (Susan Ariel Rainbow Kennedy) was broke, she stood on a street corner and said, "Miracle find me now," and six $100 bills blew down the street and into her hands. (True story.) It was possible that Dennis could continue on his sabbatical, and everything would be just hunky-dory. It was also possible that if he didn't start focusing his attention again on his business, he might lose the business and with it, his primary revenue stream. If he ran out of money and had no food, no shelter, and nobody else who could give him food or shelter (an unlikely scenario given how many people loved him, including me), then his safety might be threatened. In present time, though, he was able to pay for his basic needs.

After this, I asked Dennis to try and tune in to what his fear might have to say to him. With the guidance of his Inner Pilot

Light, could he sense what the fear was telling him about places where he was stuck, or where he needed to grow? He said:

> *Sometimes I feel my highest self taking over, but when I'm in my smallest self, I feel like I'm at the mercy of this negative current that is bigger than me, like I'm at the will of this animal, and there's no way of escaping it, no way of taking authority over my own life. I feel trapped in this prison, like I can't change the course of this trapped life. I feel like it's dragging me down every time I start to lift myself up, like it's a dark river pulling me underwater, and I can't do anything about it. When I'm in this state of mind, I feel very limited, like I can't create any good ideas and everything seems negative. I feel like a helpless victim, even though I know this kind of thinking isn't helpful. It completely paralyzes me and makes my world extremely small. Even though I know I'm not really a victim, I don't know how to get out. In my body, my breathing feels very shallow, like someone is sitting on my chest. I feel this gripping in my stomach. I feel like something is stuck in my throat and wrapped around my neck, like I'm carrying my luggage on my neck and I don't know how to escape. Because I can't stand feeling this way, I'll do anything to feel better, unaware of the motivation. I'll seek out casual sex. I'll drink alcohol or eat potato chips. I'll call my friends, the ones I know will tell me I'm great. I'm always seeking confirmation that I'm worthy of love. Even just going out on the street with this unworthy sensation, I realize I smile at random people, waiting for someone to smile back at me and give me a feeling of worthiness. If someone smiles at me, I'll feel better for a while. But if they don't smile back or if they ignore my kind gesture, I can get very angry and aggressive. It pushes all my buttons and I feel so small. There's this whole other part of me that knows it's all a lie. I'm trying to figure out how to hear and trust that voice instead. But it's so hard when this voice is so vicious and so loud.*

When Dennis focused all of his attention on the voice of his Small Self, letting it point to what was in need of healing within him, he was finally able to distance himself from the voice and see it for what it was—a critical, self-loathing tyrant without an ounce of optimism, leaving no space at all for any imagination. When false fear is running the show, the creative mind gets paralyzed. Fearful ruminations diminish creativity and shrink your perception of what's possible. But once the Small Self calms down, it's easier to tap into the part of the imagination that, instead of focusing on imagined disaster, can imagine creative solutions.

By realizing that he was not this voice, that he was actually the consciousness witnessing this vicious voice, Dennis was able to start to look at his situation more objectively. He realized that it wasn't unreasonable to start creatively problem solving about how he might generate revenue in the future. He has a publishing background, so he brainstormed how he might utilize what he loves and what he's good at to generate revenue. He dreamed of using his gifts as a scientist and publisher to explore the intersection of science and spirituality. He also saw himself writing a book, teaching workshops, and engaging in some sort of spiritual healing work. He sensed that learning about the healing arts in Peru might help him learn more about the new career his Inner Pilot Light envisioned. New possibilities were starting to open up where before he had been shut down.

COURAGE-CULTIVATING EXERCISE #2

What Can Fear Teach You?

1. Make a list of false fears that you're ruminating on right now.

2. Choose the first fear on your list, close your eyes, and take a moment to tap into your Inner Pilot Light. Breathe deeply and notice any areas of gripping, especially tightness in the belly or chest. Use the breath to breathe space into these areas and see if they loosen up. Expand your belly. Open your heart. Call in whatever it is you trust, whether it's God, the angels, the Universe, or a deity you identify with, or call on your own Inner Pilot Light directly.

3. **Ask what messages of healing your fear is try-
    ing to communicate.** What might this fear have to
    teach you about your personal and spiritual growth?
    Where might you have blind spots in need of illumi-
    nating? Where are you stuck? How can this fear be
    a blessing?

4. **Make note of whatever messages come through,
    since you'll be addressing these in Part Three of the
    book.**

YOU CAN FREE YOURSELF

It might feel extraordinarily hard to let your fear help heal
you when you're staring at mounting debt, you're responsible for
the needs of your children, your life is threatened because of a
health crisis, or you're losing the love of your life. You may feel like
only rich people have the luxury of following their dreams and
making brave choices. You may think you're not smart enough /
young enough / attractive enough / wealthy enough / motivated
enough / [fill in the blank] enough to do what your heart is guiding you to do. But you'd be mistaken if you believed the lies of
your Small Self. Cultivating courage doesn't require a fat bank account, perfect health, a genius IQ, or being footloose without a
spouse or children. Even those who feel most trapped can tap into
the kind of courage that gives them the strength to follow their
truth, rather than their fear. As part of my research for this book,
I had the opportunity to interview hundreds of people *just like you*
who decided to make courageous choices.

Pearl was the broke stay-at-home mother of two young children, with no schooling, no skills, and no job, but she found the
courage to end her unhappy marriage, even though she had no
idea how she would survive as a single mother with no money.
April, whom you've met, was a childhood sexual abuse survivor who grew up to be a badass bodyguard, until she decided to

abandon the security of her career because she knew it was only making her more afraid. Kevin was governed by the strict rules of a religious cult, frightened of what would happen if he violated the rules and escaped, but he found within himself a fortitude he didn't know he had and managed to break away. Martha wrote and published a tell-all memoir, exposing the truth about her experience with the Mormon church, even amidst death threats from the church community.

Kathleen was diagnosed with uterine cancer, and her doctor insisted that she undergo a hysterectomy, but everything in Kathleen's intuition told her she would die if she got the surgery, so she faced enormous fear and decided to decline. Martin, who was working as a pastor in a fundamentalist Christian church, came out of the closet about his homosexuality because he just couldn't betray his own truth anymore. Brian had been sexually molested as a child, and the abuse had wreaked havoc on his relationships, his sex life, his professional life, and his self-esteem, but he chose to overcome his fears of facing his past and undergo intensive therapy in order to face the beast that was ruining his life so he could finally be happy. Sally had been afraid to stand up for what she believed at work, fearing dismissal if she spoke her truth, but after years of feeling like she was selling her soul, she finally stood up to her boss.

These people don't have anything you don't have too. They didn't have any less fear than you do, and there's nothing special about them that made them choose courageous action. The voices of their false fears were just as vicious as the voices that tell you you don't have what it takes to be brave. What you need to understand is that while this voice can awaken you to what needs to be healed in your life, you don't have to let it run your life anymore. Don't be one of those people who squanders this one wild and precious life because you're taking orders from your false fear without letting it heal you. Consider this your official invitation to start trusting your Inner Pilot Light instead.

FIND YOUR STILLNESS

If you're able to distance yourself from the voice of your Small Self, you'll find that there's a place behind that voice that's very, very still and peaceful. This inner vastness of calm allows you to find your stillness even in the midst of the most chaotic circumstances. In the Find Your Calling teleclass program that Martha Beck, Amy Ahlers, and I teach, Martha leads a guided meditation that has you imagine that you're in a hurricane just above a turbulent ocean. The wind is whipping, the lightning is striking, the waves are crashing, and you're getting thrashed around by the turbulence. You then let yourself drop just beneath the surface of the ocean. From this perspective, you're still crashing around in the waves and you can look up through the surface and see the flashes of lightning, but you're underwater, so you're protected from the wind and the noise. If you dive deeper, you can go beyond the movement of the waves, and you can no longer see the flashes of lightning, and things start to get very still. Go deeper still and the ocean starts to get dark and quiet. Keep going, down, down, down until you get to the very bottom of the ocean, where you can settle into the ocean floor like you're an anchor. From this place in the ocean floor, you can be totally still. Sense your stillness. Feel the inner quiet. Nothing has changed on the surface. The hurricane is still there, with the crashing waves and wind and lightning and noise. But down at the ocean floor, it can't touch you.

There's a place inside of you that is just like this ocean floor. Your outside world can be total chaos. Maybe someone you love just died. Maybe you lost your job or got divorced. Maybe you're filing for bankruptcy or facing a cancer diagnosis. Your world might be falling apart on the outside, triggering all of your false fears. But somewhere inside of yourself, there is a place of stillness you can always access, even if you really do have a gun to your head.

Accessing this place of absolute stillness requires being in the present moment, and in this place of stillness, fear doesn't exist, not even true fear. When you're in this state of consciousness, even the death of a loved one—even your own death—doesn't scare you. You're so still and so present that you trust that, even if you die, all is well.

If you could rest in this place of stillness, with all of your attention only on the present moment, like *The Power of Now* author Eckhart Tolle did after his spiritual enlightenment, you would have one version of The Fear Cure. Focusing on what's happening right now and tuning out your Small Self, rather than projecting into the future or remembering the past, can be a potent courage-cultivating strategy. If your mind is free of thoughts, there's no false fear. End of story.

Imagine if your mind was simply still. This wouldn't mean you would lose the capacity for intellectual thought. If you needed to think in order to creatively problem solve, all of your faculties would function fully. But in between cognitive tasks, your mind would quiet down, allowing you to rest in the stillness of the present moment, where peace always lives, even in times of turmoil. The majority of our thoughts focus on fantasizing about what we want, scheming about how to get what we want, fearing what we don't want, and strategizing about how to avoid what we don't want. It's no wonder we don't feel peaceful! But there's a whole other way to live if you're willing to loosen your grip on what you want and create space between you and your fears. When you're able to stay in present time, focused only on the sensory input of what you currently see, hear, smell, taste, and feel, you'll find you get a vacation from your thoughts, and you're likely to experience peace.

While it's possible to experience this kind of peace as the result of a rapid awakening that brings you into present time instantly, most of us aren't Eckhart Tolle, at least not yet. For most of us, quieting the mind and becoming fully present is a process that requires awareness of how your Small Self operates. Once you distance yourself enough to notice how the Small Self threatens to spoil your *right now,* you can refocus your attention on what is happening in the moment and rest in the peace of the present.

COURAGE-CULTIVATING EXERCISE #3

A Meditation for Presence

1. Find a comfortable place to sit, close your eyes, and start by focusing on your breath.

2. When thoughts inevitably appear, notice the thoughts, without judgment, and let the thoughts pass through like clouds in the sky, without attaching to them. If you find yourself thinking of something in the past, call it out—"Hello, remembering." If you find yourself fantasizing about the future, notice it, too—"Hello, planning." Then come back to the breath.

3. Look for the still point between thoughts. See how long your mind can be silent between thoughts. When you notice your mind drifting off, bring it back to the breath like you're training a beloved puppy.

4. See if you can extend the gap between your thoughts. Begin to rest in the stillness of the space between thoughts. With practice, you'll find that you can rest longer and longer between thoughts.

This kind of meditation practice grants you insight into how busy the mind can be, helping you come into present time and dissociate from the kinds of thoughts that create unnecessary suffering. With practice, the space between your thoughts increases, and you're better equipped to be the witness of your Small Self, rather than at its mercy. By learning to take the position of witness to your thoughts, you discover that your thoughts are not YOU. You are the consciousness witnessing your thoughts, but they don't define you. They're just the voice of your Small Self. If you identify with them and let them dictate your decisions, you'll only create your own suffering. But if you can view this stream of thought from the witness position, you can filter out the helpful messages within it and ditch the rest, allowing yourself to relax in the peaceful quiet that arises when the Small Self's chatter drops into the background.

When you stop focusing on your thoughts about the past and the future, focusing instead on what is happening in present time, you'll realize that pain is inevitable, but most of your unnecessary suffering is caused by your resistance to what is. If you can just accept whatever is happening in the present moment, without making it wrong or trying to change it, you can be with the pain without spiraling into the suffering. Once you drop the resistance and stop identifying with the stories you make up about the negative events in your life, something loosens, and it's easier to find peace, even in the midst of painful events.

This "find your stillness" approach to dealing with fear can be sought along the path of many Eastern spiritual practices. A daily meditation practice can bring you deeper into the vastness of your inner stillness, which is a prerequisite to hearing and interpreting the guidance of your Inner Pilot Light, a key part of the Six Steps to Cultivating Courage that you'll learn in Part Three. Finding your stillness will also help you with what you'll learn and practice in Part Two of this book, which is all about helping you identify and heal beliefs that may predispose you to letting false fear run the show. As you learn to focus on the awareness of the breath and the body, you are thrust into present time, which helps you move out of the mind and into the now. This Eastern way of dealing with fear may be right up your alley, and you may want to include daily meditation, yoga, the practice of presence, and other such practices in your Prescription for Courage. From this place of stillness, you'll have the opportunity to shift from a fear-based to a trust-based worldview that guides you to a state of inner peacefulness, rather than inner reactivity and the need to control life. When you can get still, you'll be able to simply accept, rather than resist, what is. In the place that allows you to accept reality, even when reality isn't going the way you like, you'll also find the gateway to your courage. In order to fully activate this courage, you'll need not only inner stillness but also new, courage-cultivating beliefs that help your Small Self feel calm and safe so you can take brave risks without your Small Self freaking out. By unearthing and healing the root causes of false fear, you will find your brave.

ROOT CAUSES OF FALSE FEAR

I've studied fear from a range of perspectives that all inform the work we're doing in this book, from mystical religious traditions to Western psychology to the lessons of *A Course in Miracles,* and when I examine fear through the lens of all of these influences, I see that much of our false fear stems from limiting beliefs that make up our worldview. When you're mindful of the thoughts that drive your decision making, you can make the choice to shift from fear-inducing beliefs that trigger false fear to courage-cultivating beliefs that make you brave. So an essential part of letting fear cure you is examining the thoughts that make you scared so you can shift to thoughts that induce peace and engender courage instead.

All false fear arises from thought, and in my experience with clients and the people I interviewed, as well as in my own experience, almost all false fear thoughts stem from four myths that many of us mistakenly adopt as truth. These fear-inducing limiting beliefs, which I call the Four Fearful Assumptions, represent the dominant worldview of our modern Western culture and lead us to experience a lot of unnecessary suffering. See if any of the following beliefs sound familiar to you.

FOUR FEARFUL ASSUMPTIONS

Uncertainty is unsafe.
I can't handle losing what I cherish.
It's a dangerous world.
I am all alone.

The Four Fearful Assumptions are merely thoughts, but your Small Self most likely has adopted these cultural beliefs as gospel truth—as so many of us have. Because we believe we can't feel safe in the face of uncertainty, we conclude that we must pursue safety, security, and certainty at all costs, even if the cost is our health and happiness. Because we believe we can't handle losing what we cherish, we try to vigilantly guard against loss, even when doing so makes us cling to what we just can't keep. Because we grow up believing we live in a dangerous world, often because of what we learned in childhood, we conclude that it's up to us to ward off poverty, violence, illness, pain, rejection, and abandonment. And because we assume we are separate, distinct individuals navigating this dangerous world alone, the primal survival instincts of our tribal species get triggered and convince us we are vulnerable to injury or death. When this is our dominant worldview, it's no wonder we wind up feeling very frightened. We simply have too much to lose, and *we are not okay with this.* Deep down, we're terrified that we simply cannot handle it if our greatest fears come true.

Yet the Four Fearful Assumptions are relatively recent phenomena in the history of our species. By all measures, primitive human beings used to live in a much more dangerous and uncertain world than we do now. Mothers and children regularly died in childbirth. Everyone and everything was vulnerable to the elements. Living quarters could be easily devastated by natural disasters. Infectious diseases could wipe out a whole tribe. Death and loss were commonplace. People still grieved when they lost what they loved, but they survived and grew from the loss, receiving comfort from the tribal mythology and rituals and communion with the spirit realm, which imbued such loss with meaning and purpose. Their worldview helped them handle the kinds of hardships we can't even fathom.

Not until the scientific revolution did the driving need for knowledge and certainty overtake our willingness to live in the realm of mythology, metaphor, and mystery. The quest for certainty initially helped us feel safe because we began to understand more about how the world works. This knowledge allowed us some understanding of science, so we no longer believed we were at the whim of uncertain, unexplainable, unpredictable forces, the way indigenous cultures often did. But this craving for certainty came with a dark side. We lost our tolerance for uncertainty and loss, and this led us to conclude that we lived all alone in a dangerous world.

As modern life evolved, we shifted from a culture that perceived ourselves to be intricately interlinked beings in constant communion with nature into a culture where the dominant worldview is that we are separate, distinct, carbon-based life forms whose consciousness exists only in our brains. Indigenous cultures believed everything to be connected—not just all humans or even all animals, but water, the ocean, the mountains, even the weather. Today, we have come to believe that we are connected to nothing, which is one reason the survival of the planet is now at risk. Fortunately, since our culture's fear-inducing beliefs are just that—beliefs—we can take the opportunity to question our fears and heal our thoughts.

THE FOUR COURAGE-CULTIVATING TRUTHS

So what can we do to transform our relationship with false fear? We can make a conscious choice to replace fearful thoughts with thoughts that comfort, heal, and help us feel safe. To use a simple example, if your thought is *I'm not good enough,* it's helpful to recognize that this is just a thought—one that limits you—and ask yourself what might be an alternative to this thought, something to empower and free you instead.

In *Loving What Is,* Byron Katie teaches "The Work," which is based on four questions that help you turn around a limiting belief into a more genuine truth. Sometimes the turnaround is an affirmation that is the direct opposite of the limiting belief. For example, the turnaround of *I'm not good enough* might be *I am enough.* But often, the turnaround is deeper and more complex than the simple opposite of the limiting belief. When we apply a similar sort of "turnaround" logic to the Four Fearful Assumptions, we can replace these limiting beliefs with a set of empowering beliefs that I call the Four Courage-Cultivating Truths.

FOUR COURAGE-CULTIVATING TRUTHS

Truth #1: Uncertainty is the gateway to possibility.
Truth #2: Loss is natural and can lead to growth.
Truth #3: It's a purposeful universe.
Truth #4: We are all One.

Making this shift from the Four Fearful Assumptions to the Four Courage-Cultivating Truths is less of a cognitive process and more of an intuitive one. I will offer your cognitive mind evidence that the Four Courage-Cultivating Truths can be trusted, but your cognitive mind will keep trying to talk you out of believing them. Your cognitive mind is not your friend when it comes to letting fear heal you. Although it's trying to be helpful, when it comes to false fear, your cognitive mind can hurt you more than it can help because it tends to be governed by your Small Self, rather than by your Inner Pilot Light. This is where the intuitive argument comes in. Your Inner Pilot Light governs your intuition, and it already knows that the Four Courage-Cultivating Truths can be trusted. So the real shift happens when you learn to trust this part of you.

The worldview I'll be presenting to you in the next four chapters is not something I just randomly pulled out of my black doctor's bag. I'll be providing your cognitive mind with all the evidence I can find to support this worldview, which is based on the Four Courage-Cultivating Truths. Some of this evidence comes from high-quality clinical trials published in the peer-reviewed scientific literature. Some comes from the experience of people whose stories have been published in other reputable books. Some evidence comes from the stories of people I've interviewed personally, and other evidence is drawn from my own personal experience. In the next four chapters, I will be inviting both your cognitive mind and your intuition to consider embracing these truths, so you can cement your new beliefs into a courage-cultivating worldview that makes you feel safer and braver.

When you believe the Four Courage-Cultivating Truths, you're on your way to living a more courageous life. Once you come into right relationship with uncertainty, you're able to face uncertainty with excitement and curiosity, rather than fear. When you accept the inevitability of loss, loss can help you grow. Once you realize you're always being guided by a Universal Intelligence that's purposeful, rather than dangerous, you start to trust that everything's happening for a reason, even if you don't always understand why. When you really sense that we are all part of a collective consciousness, you stop feeling so cosmically lonely and start realizing we're all connected, and this helps you become brave enough to live out your life purpose. When you shift from abiding by the Four Fearful Assumptions and start letting the Four Courage-Cultivating Truths guide your actions, you heal yourself and bless the world.

CHAPTER 4

UNCERTAINTY IS *the* GATEWAY *to* POSSIBILITY

*People have a hard time letting go of their suffering. Out of a
fear of the unknown, they prefer suffering that is familiar.*

— THICH NHAT HANH

Every day, Kris Carr wakes up not knowing whether today
could be her last. We all do, technically. Any one of us could
die today. But for Kris, it's more in her face. Kris was in her early
30s when she was diagnosed with a rare type of stage 4 cancer for
which there is no cure. Radiation and chemotherapy don't work,
and the only surgical options include transplanting her tumor-
ridden organs, which still doesn't address the microscopic cancer
cells that line her blood vessels.

When Kris was diagnosed, she was told to do whatever she
could to support her immune system, so she embarked upon a radical journey of self-healing, which included switching to a largely

raw, vegan diet but also included spiritual practices and other life-style changes. Regardless, she was informed that she would prob-ably die within ten years. Kris made it her mission to prove that you could be "crazy" and "sexy" and still thrive with cancer. She turned her cancer journey into a documentary film, *Crazy Sexy Cancer,* and has since inspired millions with her message about how to be a "cancer thriver."

Along the way, Kris had to deal with a lot of understandable fear. Her cancer was diagnosed on Valentine's Day, so every Febru-ary 14, she would get a CT scan that assessed the size of her tumors, an understandably fear-invoking annual event. She never knew what the scan would find. As it turned out, every year, the tumors were the same. They hadn't grown, but they hadn't shrunk.

After a decade of fearing something she couldn't control, something in Kris finally shifted and she allowed her fear to point to one thing that needed healing in her relationship to her cancer—her tendency to resist it. After ten years of hoping her cancer would one day go away, she decided to let go of her attachment to a cure. Instead, she chose to accept her cancer and to thrive in the face of the ultimate uncertainty. On her eleventh Valentine's Day anniversary, Kris got the good news. For the first time ever, her tumors had actually shrunk.

Although we are always staring uncertainty in the face, few people ever have the opportunity to consciously practice making peace with uncertainty on a daily basis the way Kris Carr did. Most of us do everything within our power to avoid uncertainty, and when we do face it, we do everything we can to try to return to a state of certainty. But making peace with uncertainty may be one of the most powerful spiritual practices there is.

Immaculée Ilibagiza was also faced with daily fear and the constant threat of death. During the Rwanda genocide in 1994, Immaculée, a Tutsi, spent 91 days huddled silently together with seven other women in a Hutu pastor's cramped bathroom, not knowing from one minute to the next whether she would be found and having no idea what awaited her on the outside. A healthy 115-pound university student when she entered the bathroom, she weighed 65 pounds when she came out to discover the worst—that most of the Tutsis in her village, including almost all of her family members, had been violently murdered while she was in hiding.

Immaculée says she would have been crippled by fear, anger, and resentment had she not been in constant prayer, holding a set of rosary beads given to her by her devout Catholic father before she went into hiding. Even in the face of overwhelming evidence that we live in a dangerous world, living in constant communion with a divine force helped her find peace and solace during her confinement. Later, after she was released from the bathroom, she found herself face-to-face with a Hutu with a machete, who threatened to kill her. Instead of succumbing to fear, she stared down the man, and he let her escape, along with the other refugees who accompanied her. Years later, when she was working for the United Nations, she was given the opportunity to face the man who had murdered her mother and brother. Others expected her to spit on the man, but instead Immaculée said, "I forgive you."

Kris Carr and Immaculée Ilibagiza offer extreme examples of individuals who were able to find peace in unusually uncertain and frightening circumstances. But you can too.

I present these two examples to help us question Fearful Assumption #1: "Uncertainty is unsafe." You might argue that both Kris and Immaculée were unsafe in the face of uncertainty. After all, Kris still has stage 4 cancer, and Immaculée almost lost her life in the Rwanda genocide. But both are thriving at this point in their lives. Kris is inspiring millions of people to realize they can thrive in the face of uncertainty, rather than letting fear of the unknown stunt their growth. Immaculée is teaching the orphans of genocide to forgive those who killed their families so we can stop the cycles of revenge and violence that plague our world. I suspect both would agree with Courage-Cultivating Truth #1: "Uncertainty is the gateway to possibility." I'll bet you can think of examples in your own life when your willingness to lean into uncertain times without resistance opened a doorway into something larger. But most people don't let themselves think this way . . .

ADDICTED TO CERTAINTY

We are a culture of certainty addicts, yet the reality is that we can't know what will happen even one minute in the future. For all we know, the earth could get hit by some cosmic event that would destroy our whole planet tomorrow. *And we are simply not okay with this.* We smother our deep-seated fear of uncertainty with food, alcohol, cigarettes, excessive exercise, busyness, television, and other numbing behaviors that distract us from our discomfort with the fact that we can't control life the way we wish we could. We collect more and more things to make ourselves feel safe, and then we become even more afraid that we might lose what we've acquired. Our primary goal becomes keeping things safe and secure, even at the price of living a rich, meaningful life full of opportunities for soul growth and real connection.

Because we're so uncomfortable with uncertainty, we make up stories to comfort ourselves, stories that fluff up our sense of certainty, like "My child will never get cancer," "I'll keep my stable job forever," "A natural disaster will never threaten my life," "I'll always have plenty of money," "I won't die until I'm a hundred years old," or "My beloved will always love me." On some level, we know that our stories of certainty are nothing more than illusion. These stories we tell ourselves are only thoughts, yet we cling to these thoughts, which are fueled by underlying fears, and we become emotionally overwrought if the certainty of our stories is threatened. Many people will sleep through life in this way until what we fear most happens and tragedy hits. A life-threatening illness strikes. A loved one dies. You're fired from your seemingly stable job. Financial ruin befalls you. Such life changes shake you awake only to reveal that it's hard to go back to sleep, now that you're aware that certainty is nothing but an illusion.

How you deal with uncertainty tends to differ depending on how you approach new situations. Rachel Naomi Remen, M.D., taught me that we each have a part of ourselves that we trust the most—our "frontrunner." When we come into a new situation, especially an uncertain one, we send the most trusted part of ourselves in first to check out and validate the scene. The cognitive person sends in the cognitive mind. You ask, *Who's there? How reliable are they? What does the data say? Does this make sense? How does it work? Can I explain it? Is there a mechanism I can prove?*

But maybe it's not the cognitive mind that you trust. Maybe you trust your heart or your intuition. When you send that in as the frontrunner, you might ask, *What's the vibe in here? How does it feel? Are people loving? Are they connecting? Are they competing? Does it feel aligned to be here? Do I belong?*

The cognitive mind, while useful when it comes to solving cognitive tasks, is also the birthplace of the scared voice of your Small Self. This may not make sense to the mind, since the mind thinks of itself as the smart, adult, trustworthy voice. But while it's true that the intellect comes from the cognitive mind, fear stems from thoughts arising in the mind as well. Your Inner Pilot Light, on the other hand, resides in your heart and your intuition. Your Small Self craves certainty, but your Inner Pilot Light is just as comfortable with the unknown as with the known. It doesn't require certainty in order to feel at peace.

We all have within us both parts, but many people in our culture trust the cognitive mind more than we trust intuition, so we give the cognitive mind more power to validate our experiences. This creates a problem, because the smaller part of you (your cognitive mind, or Small Self) cannot easily validate a larger part of you (your heart and intuition, or Inner Pilot Light). You can validate the conclusions of the cognitive mind with intuition, but you can't do the opposite. You get stuck, because the cognitive mind craves certainty. It will always seek safety, security, and comfort, even at the expense of personal integrity, alignment, adventure, and joy.

What determines whether someone is a "cognitive validator" or driven by intuition instead? As children, when we face recurrent uncertainty and don't feel safe, we tend to "go cognitive." We start to crave explanations, a sense of control, rational thinking, and a feeling of certainty. It makes us feel like we have some control over our uncertain world. But "going cognitive" cuts us off from our capacity to lean into uncertainty with curiosity, wonder, even awe.

Think about what you give up if you insist on certainty. You close the door on curiosity, creativity, and possibility, you cut off your openness to new things, and you miss out on the excitement of being a perpetual student. As Rachel Naomi Remen says, when we take this stance, "We trade mystery for mastery and lose a sense of aliveness and possibility."

Traditionally, I have been a cognitive validator. Twelve years of medical education drilled into me the importance of valuing the rational, logical cognitive mind above all else. I always felt most comfortable when I could rationally explain how things worked. I valued science, with its detailed explanations about the nature of things. I felt uneasy in the presence of things I couldn't explain. Yet something started to loosen in the wake of my Perfect Storm.

MY PERFECT STORM

Prior to my Perfect Storm, I was slogging along in what might have looked like a perfect, predictable, stable life, but this security came at a price. What others didn't know was that my life was unraveling from the inside out. I had the "dream job" working as a full-time OB-GYN physician, making a cushy six-figure salary that allowed me certain luxuries, like an ocean-view house in San Diego, fancy European cars, and vacations in Hawaii. My job afforded me a certain position of respect and status in society, and I was admired by my peers as a skilled, conscientious doctor who really cared about her patients. My personal life also looked great on paper: I was married to a kind, intelligent, loving man, we were about to have our first child, and I had a lot of friends. By the age of 35, I had achieved everything I was taught to believe would make me happy, which is why I felt guilty and ungrateful for feeling so desperately unhappy, like I'd somehow sold my soul in exchange for the "perfect life."

For years, I had been feeling an inner restlessness I couldn't quite explain. Why was I not happy? I had everything society says you should have in order to live the good life. I tried focusing on gratitude. I had so much to be grateful for. Surely, if I focused on being grateful, I could find the spring in my step that would allow me to navigate the next 30 years in my high-pressure career until I could finally retire at 65 and really enjoy life.

But gratitude wasn't working, and I was often waking up at 2 A.M. in tears. I tried to ignore my unhappiness, busying myself with my satisfying career as a doctor, beginning a successful professional art career on the side, and drinking wine in the evenings to take the edge off my growing feeling of uneasiness. But my efforts to distract myself weren't working. My body was betraying me, with the laundry list of chronic illnesses I faced mounting as the years passed. By the time I was 35, I was taking seven medications for a whole host of chronic health conditions that were only getting worse with treatment. I should have predicted that the Universe was about to call my bluff, but I got blindsided when my wake-up call finally came.

When I was six months pregnant with my daughter, my mother called me to tell me that my father was making up words. When she put him on the phone, he told me he needed to go to a "travel one llama center." I knew something was very wrong and, thinking he was having a stroke, I told Mom to take him to the emergency room right away. When they did a CT scan, they found an enormous brain tumor in Dad's temporal lobe, and after a further workup, they found other tumors all over his body. A biopsy of a liver tumor confirmed the diagnosis of metastatic melanoma. My beloved father, who was only 59, was given three months to live.

Almost exactly three months later, I gave birth to my daughter, Siena, by C-section. I was recovering from surgery when my father and mother flew out to San Diego to meet their granddaughter. A course of whole brain radiation had failed to shrink my father's tumor, and Dad's doctors predicted that the end was near, so my parents rented a beach house, where Hospice brought in a hospital bed, and my father prepared to die while I nursed my daughter and the incision on my belly.

My brother Chris and my sister Keli both live out of town, so they flew in to be with my father in his final days. When healthy

33-year-old Chris arrived, he wound up in the emergency room in full-blown liver failure as a rare side effect of the antibiotic Zithromax, which he was taking for a sinus infection. That same week, my beloved 16-year-old dog, Ariel, died. Then, exactly two weeks after I had given birth to my daughter, we lost Dad. It was the most traumatic two weeks of my life, and it changed everything. I suddenly realized that certainty was merely an illusion, and having awoken from the dream state, I found myself staring, terrified, into the vast mystery of the uncertain. I wasn't sure I could handle it.

A series of uncertain tragedies, like the ones that made up my Perfect Storm, have a tendency to affect people in one of two ways. Either you shut down, demanding even more certainty, guarding even more against the unknown, fortifying your cognitive mind and instructing it to be on high alert, or the absurdity of life hits you so hard that you're knocked to the ground. The seeming meaninglessness of life tears you apart and you find yourself feeling lonelier than you thought it possible to feel. You're driven to the edge of insanity with despair. And then, just as you're losing faith in the cognitive mind, something bigger reaches up to meet you in your devastation. In this annihilated state, you may surprise yourself with a strength you never knew you had, one that allows you to do what you never thought you could—accept the unacceptable. What you're really doing here is letting fear cure you.

This ability to accept the unacceptable may only last for a few minutes, but when it happens, it leaves a crack in the shell of who you thought you were. Through this crack, there's an opportunity for the light of who you really are to shine through, often for the first time since infancy. Once this crack appears, once you have even one moment in which you see your true nature, you can never unsee it. You may turn your back on it. You may deny it. But you will never be the same, because you have glimpsed another state of consciousness, one far vaster than the limited view of yourself that has dominated your sense of identity for so long.

THE SMALL SELF'S QUEST FOR CERTAINTY

If we let it, uncertainty brings us face-to-face with the nature of the Small Self. One of the reasons we cling to the illusion of certainty is because it gives the Small Self the false sense that we're in control. Because the Small Self is the part of you that has an investment in maintaining your self-image and your worldview, the Small Self likes to be certain. The Small Self has a story about the kind of person you are, the kind of person you're not, what you're good at, what you're not good at, what you're capable of achieving, what you're not, what you believe, what you don't. The Small Self also has strong ideas about how the world works—what's right, what's wrong, what's real, what's not, what's possible, what's impossible, what's sane, and what's crazy. The Small Self doesn't like questions that don't have certain answers, and it's willing to sacrifice mystery, wonder, awe, and possibility in order to fit everything into orderly boxes.

In *Falling into Grace,* spiritual teacher Adyashanti teaches that we begin as a vast inner space of quiet awareness. Then we are given a name, a gender, a series of rules for what's "right" and what's "wrong," and ideas about our place in the world. As we accumulate experiences, we build upon these ideas to solidify our self-image and our worldview. Some of us have a negative self-image, filled with painful thoughts about how we're not good enough. Some of us have a positive self-image. Whether you feel superior or inferior, more worthy or less worthy, smarter than or stupider than, prettier than or uglier than, it's all a story. These ideas are nothing more than thoughts, yet we're so identified with them that we forget who we really are—pure consciousness free of the limitations of thought.

Everything in modern society feeds the Small Self. We shore it up, make up stories about it, pick out its outfits, and dress it up in a false aura of perfection. If anything or anybody challenges this image of who we are and how the world works, we get very uncomfortable. We wind up wearing masks because we're afraid of disrupting the image we hope to project in the world, but then we wind up feeling like frauds because we're not being honest about who we really are. Our quest for certainty creates suffering because, as much as we're afraid of having our certainty shattered, we know in our hearts it's even more tragic if we die with the song of who we are left unsung.

My patient Heidi showed up at my office one day in a total tizzy because she'd just had sex with her new boyfriend and failed to disclose to this guy, whom she really liked, that she had herpes. She asked for my help. How could she rectify what she had done and protect her boyfriend without losing face?

Heidi said, "Dr. Rankin, you don't understand. I'm a person of integrity. I don't do things like this." She hung her head, unable to make eye contact with me.

I said, "What if, instead of being certain that you are a person of integrity, you're simply curious about the kind of person you really are? Maybe you're a person of integrity. Maybe you're not. Maybe what you believe about yourself is true sometimes and not true other times. Would you be willing to let go of your story of who you think you are?"

I felt safe taking the risk to say what I did to Heidi because I know how dedicated she is to her personal and spiritual growth, and I knew she'd accept my challenge with love, which she did. Heidi got it. She went home and confessed to her boyfriend what she had withheld. He chose to start prophylactic treatment that could reduce his likelihood of getting herpes. The two were still together two years later when I saw Heidi for her Pap smear.

The Small Self tends to take conflicting views of who we are. We inflate ourselves by making up stories about how noble, smart, and full of integrity we are. Then we deflate ourselves with stories about how worthless we are when we fail to live up to those inflated ideas, letting down ourselves and others. The Small Self is always comparing us, judging us as either inferior to those we admire or superior to those we judge as "less than." The truth of who we really are usually lies somewhere in the middle, where we're able to witness our true magnificence from a place of humility and curiosity, where we are no better than or worse than anyone else, where we simply are who we are as we each walk our own unique path of soul growth. If we're willing to simply be curious, our true nature starts to reveal itself. It can be painfully uncomfortable to put everything you think you know up for question, but if you're willing to be curious, life can be your teacher. That's where the real magic lies.

LIFE AS THE TEACHER

As Rachel Naomi Remen pointed out in the Medicine for the Soul teleclass we taught together, life can be the teacher, if only we let it. As children, as soon as we start preschool, we make up a story about how the teachers know it all, and we, as students, know nothing. We admire these teachers and long to be like them. Clearly, it is more valuable to know than not to know. Not knowing makes you small and weak. Knowing makes you big and powerful. We come to the conclusion that the more we know, the better our lives will be. This leads us to become intolerant of that which we don't know. We start to value certainty at all costs. We come to believe that it's better to be a knower than a learner.

When Rachel was in second grade, she told her mother she loved knowing things, but she hated learning things. When asked what she wanted to be when she grew up, she said, full of confidence, "An expert." But when Rachel grew up, she realized that the true wisdom lies in being the learner, rather than the knower. Sure, there is knowledge we can acquire in school, from books, and through our teachers. But there is something priceless that lies beyond knowledge. The willingness to be humble and curious, to simply wonder whether something is true, opens a doorway to possibility. It frees us from the limits of certainty and allows life to become our own mystery school.

Life as the teacher shows up in a variety of ways. Your children may be your teachers. The homeless guy on the street can be your teacher. Heartbreak can be your teacher. Abuse can be your teacher. Fear can be your teacher. Many of the gifts life has to teach us live not in the realm of the certain, but in the uncertain. A willingness to let life be your teacher requires a certain humility, but we are all capable of becoming learners if we're willing to not know. Whether you're the President of the United States or the dean of Harvard or a kindergartener, life can be your teacher, if only you'll let it. It will tend to point to the places where your craving for certainty has made you the most blind.

This is what happened to me during my Perfect Storm. I was humbled by the stunning series of losses I experienced. My Small Self was still defending against uncertainty, but the crack left by my Perfect Storm began to widen, and it left everything in my life open to question. I suddenly woke up from the illusion of certainty that I would live to be a hundred and nothing I cherished would ever be lost. I realized that just as my father had suddenly been given only three months to live, the same thing could happen to me at any point. When I asked myself whether I would be living the same life if I knew I had only three months left to live, the answer was a resounding "Hell, no."

I wound up making the difficult decision to quit my stable job in conventional medicine. Doing so would require selling my house and moving to the country, where the cost of living was lower. My daughter was only eight months old, and I was the sole breadwinner, since my husband, Matt, wasn't working outside the home. I finally got up the nerve to tell my partners I was leaving my practice to embark into the vast unknown without a safety net or even a backup plan. That's when Matt cut two fingers off his left hand with a table saw. After eight hours in surgery, a microsurgeon was able to reattach Matt's fingers, but he warned us that Matt would need further surgery to make the fingers functional. With that kind of preexisting condition, I had to postpone leaving my job. The pain of staying put after I had already made the decision to leave was almost unbearable. I felt trapped. I questioned my decision. Was it a sign I had made the wrong choice? Or was my commitment simply being tested? Finally, after months of Matt's surgeries, physical therapy, and recovery, and enduring the feeling that I simply couldn't stay in my job one more day, no matter what the cost, I quit.

Between medical bills, leaving my job, buying my freedom by paying my medical malpractice "tail"—insurance that would cover me, once I'd left my practice, against claims of malpractice in the past—and paying for living expenses while neither my husband nor I were working, we went from owning our house with plenty of money in a retirement account to renting with over $200,000 in debt. I came face-to-face with uncertainty and all the fears it brought up—and I let fear and life teach me. My Perfect Storm and the choices I made in its wake became the first in a series of initiation rites that thrust me onto the spiritual path. I went from feeling terrified of the unknown to seeing the unknown as a potential gift. Maybe instead of being afraid of what I didn't know, I could not only accept it; I could even allow it to excite me. Instead of viewing the unknown as a personal failure, I could see it as a gift from the Universe, an opportunity to learn, if only I was willing to be humble enough to seek out the lesson.

What I discovered is that the flip side of the fear of uncertainty is the excitement of possibility. Instead of fearing "I don't know," you start embracing "I don't know" with a sense of adventure, because when you don't know what the future holds, anything can happen. Such a perspective flies in the face of all of our cultural conditioning. The cognitive validator in us always wants to know "how" and "why." But as Rachel said to me when I kept asking "how" and "why," "Perhaps understanding how and why is the booby prize."

Something magical happens when you stop trying to control every aspect of your life and commit to letting life be your teacher, even when things aren't going your way. When you're willing to release your grip on certainty and lean into the mystery of the unknown, life can start to delight you. You grow. You transform. You're ready to move past the false fears that hold you back and lean into uncertainty from a place of faith.

MOVING FROM FEAR TO FREEDOM

When we're willing to view life as the teacher, even in the midst of uncertainty, a journey begins. This journey—some might call it the spiritual path—challenges us to shift from fear of uncertainty to trusting life in the face of that which we can't know and don't understand. After interviewing many people about what they'd learned on their own spiritual journeys, I discovered that the journey from fear to freedom, which is all about coming into right relationship with uncertainty, is a predictable journey, one that many have traveled before you and many will travel after you. As you read through the five phases, consider where you are on your own journey.

THE JOURNEY FROM FEAR TO FREEDOM

Phase 1: Unconscious Fear of Uncertainty. *I stay in my comfort zone and avoid the unknown at all costs.* What I don't know feels dangerous, but I'm not conscious of how uncomfortable I am with uncertainty. I never get close enough to the unknown to really feel it. I do not act without a sense of certainty about the outcome. I expend a lot of energy avoiding risk.

Phase 1 Motto: "Better safe than sorry."

How to navigate Phase 1: Start becoming aware of how your inclination to cling to certainty limits your freedom. Ask yourself, "Is this working for me? Is staying in my comfort zone really protecting me?"

Phase 2: Conscious Fear of Uncertainty. *What I don't know feels dangerous, but I'm aware of the fear I feel.* Situations of uncertainty provoke feelings of anxiety, worry, and fear in me. This leads me to avoid uncertain situations and to try to control my world. But though I prefer certainty, I'm aware of how clinging to it is holding me back. I resist the unknown, but I realize it's hard to have adventures if you're always waiting to be sure of the future.

Phase 2 Motto: "The only thing certain in life is uncertainty."

How to navigate Phase 2: Be gentle with yourself as you recognize how your drive for certainty limits your possibility. Don't beat yourself up because you resist uncertainty. Pat yourself on the back for being brave enough to admit it. From a place of radical self-compassion, you will naturally begin to shift into Phase 3.

Phase 3: Uncertainty Limbo. *I don't know whether the unknown is dangerous or not.* I'm not entirely at ease with what I don't know, but I'm not resisting it, either. The unknown doesn't outright scare me, but I don't seek it out. I'm starting to sense the freedom that comes with making peace with uncertainty, so I'm willing to be cautiously curious and let my fear of the unknown teach me.

Phase 3 Motto: "I'm curious about the unknown, but I have my reservations."

How to navigate Phase 3: Question everything. Stay open. Be curious. Resist the urge to create artificial certainty in order to ease any discomfort you still feel with the unknown. If you seek out too much certainty during this phase, you're likely to allow fear to create something not quite in alignment with the full realization of what's possible. Live in limbo and do what you can to comfort yourself and find your peace.

Phase 4: Uncertainty Seduction. *Not only am I not scared by uncertainty, I'm downright attracted to it.* I realize there is more to know and the only way to know it is to lean into the unknown and explore it. To me, the unknown is not scary, it's somewhat seductive. I'm more in touch with discovering, and with the enlivenment that accompanies the discovery process, than I am with knowing. Discovery is sexier than certainty, and I'm at risk of being reckless as uncertainty seduces me. I'm so willing to entertain the unknown, to step into it and see what's there, that I don't always practice discernment. I'm willing to become an adventurer, but I have to remember not to yo-yo to the opposite end of the uncertainty spectrum.

Phase 4 Motto: "The flip side of the fear of uncertainty is the excitement of possibility."

How to navigate Phase 4: The key to Phase 4 is discernment. When the unknown becomes compelling, it can be tempting to leap blindly, but this can get you in trouble. Someone who experiences no fear in the face of the unknown is at risk of becoming reckless. Healthy behavior in Phase 4 allows you to approach uncertainty with discriminating decision making, fueled not by fear, but by the integrity of the soul and the guidance of your intuition.

Phase 5: Surrender. *I don't know, but I trust anyway.* I'm not afraid of the unknown, and I'm not seduced by it, either. I practice discernment. I sense that there is an organizing principle I may never fully understand, but I have faith that leaning in this direction is safe. Good things may happen when I lean into the unknown. Bad things may happen too. But regardless of what happens, I trust that I live in a purposeful universe and that there is meaning in all outcomes. I am simply open to wonder, and I value freedom more than I value certainty.

Phase 5 Motto: "The only way to experience life's richness is to surrender to the unknown."

How to navigate Phase 5: Enjoy! Phase 5 tends to be very peaceful, but you don't usually land there and stay there. Remaining in Phase 5 is a constant practice. If you find yourself slipping back into fear in the face of the unknown, remind yourself to trust that there are unseen forces guiding you in ways you may not understand until you look back.

Keep in mind that your journey through these five phases may not be linear. You may leap forward from one phase to the next, only to find that you regress in times of loss or trauma. Because we're often more comfortable with uncertainty in some areas of our lives than in others, you may not be in the same phase in all aspects of your life. For example, you may be in Phase 4 in your professional life and Phase 2 in your love life. Be sure not to judge yourself based on where you are. There is no "right" or "wrong" phase, and you have to trust your own timing. The reason to identify where you are on your journey is not to trigger your "not good enough" story, but simply to help guide you as you walk your own path in your own timing. Be extra gentle and compassionate with yourself as you navigate this journey from fear to freedom. As Rachel Naomi Remen says, "You can't make a rosebud open by hitting it with a hammer." Trust the process and indulge yourself with radical self-care. Know that wherever you are, you are in the right place.

ARE YOU OKAY WITH "I DON'T KNOW"?

Consider your own relationship to uncertainty. Are you willing to let life be your teacher? Are you willing to make decisions that have no certain outcome, or is fear holding you back? Are you willing to let your fear of the unknown point a finger at everything you're clinging to and need to release? Is it time to take a risk and go back to school after all these years? Is it time to take a risk in your marriage that may grow the relationship but might also threaten it? Is there enough trust in your relationship to take a risk that might deepen your sexual intimacy? Is it time to invest your money in fulfilling a lifelong dream, even though you might lose your financial security? Are you ready to finally find the courage to heal from childhood traumas? Is it time to move to the place that feels like the heart of your soul?

Life is full of opportunities to take leaps of faith. But can you be comfortable with the uncertainty that accompanies such leaps? Is it the right time? Can you make peace with—and even love—all the question marks in your life?

Rainer Maria Rilke wrote, "Be patient towards all that is unsolved in your heart. Try to love the questions themselves."

COURAGE-CULTIVATING EXERCISE #4

Practice Uncertainty

Like strengthening your biceps, changing your relationship with uncertainty requires exercise. Try a bench press for your uncertainty muscles. Push the limits of your comfort zone with activities loaded with built-in uncertainty.

- **Rejection Therapy.** Do you fear the uncertainty of facing possible rejection? Set yourself up to get rejected. Entrepreneur and professional "fearbuster" Jia Jiang was afraid of rejection, so he challenged himself with 100 Days of Rejection, during which he challenged himself to ask for things for which he expected a no. Put yourself in situations where you expect to get turned down. Notice that even when your fear of being rejected happens, you can handle it.

- **Get Lost.** Afraid of the uncertainty of an unplanned road trip? Challenge yourself to get in your car and just keep turning left. I once went on a first date with a guy who did this. We wound up eating frozen lemonade at a Little League baseball game among strangers before having to stop at a gas station to ask for directions back to where we came from. Be willing to experiment. Get adventurous. See where you end up.

- **Open Yourself to Failure.** Afraid of not knowing whether or not you'll succeed? Put yourself in situations where your success is uncertain. Take a class to learn an obscure skill you've never tried. Be willing to put yourself out there and fail. Discover that you're not good at everything, *and that this is okay.* Laugh at your failures. Celebrate how brave you were for trying. Think about how much fun you have if you go bowling when you don't know how to bowl. Imagine someone roller-skating for the first time. We don't expect children to be good at something the first time they do it, but somehow we expect this of ourselves. Try not to take yourself so seriously. Be willing to fail miserably—or not so miserably! Rather than fixating on mastery, learn to relish the excitement of trying something new.

COURAGE-CULTIVATING EXERCISE #5

Uncertainty Meditation

If you're facing an uncertain situation and finding yourself fearful, download the Prescription for Courage Kit, available for free download at TheFearCureBook.com, and listen to the Uncertainty Meditation.

CHAPTER 5

LOSS IS NATURAL
and CAN LEAD
to GROWTH

*Grief is not about forgetting; it's
about remembering with gratitude.*

— RACHEL NAOMI REMEN, M.D.

As a child, Cameron Clapp was a well-behaved identical twin, born into a large Mormon family. He and his twin, Jesse, were athletic, handsome, popular, and academically gifted. Their parents got divorced when the twins were in middle school, and the divorce sent shock waves through the family that changed Cameron into a rebellious teenager with green and blue earrings and green and blue hair. He quit caring about school and started partying every weekend, never considering how his drinking would change his life. Even getting arrested for driving under the influence at the age of 15 while "borrowing" his neighbor's minivan failed to knock Cameron off his self-destructive path.

Cameron and Jesse lived across the street from the train tracks, right next to a campground where they regularly sneaked in late at night, wearing camouflage gear, and stole hundreds of beers from the coolers of sleeping campers. As they drank into the wee hours of the night, Cameron never considered what would one day happen on those same train tracks he sat on.

Cameron was 15 years old on September 14, 2001, three days after the tragedies of September 11. He and his twin were very patriotic, planning to join the armed forces when they grew up, so when President Bush told the American people to light candles in honor of those who had fallen on September 11, Cameron and Jesse built a shrine to the victims with candles, a flag, and a spotlight before heading to a three-kegger party to help them numb the pain. They drank there until the party got busted, then they headed to a second party, where they switched from beer to hard alcohol.

Later that night, back at home, Cameron stumbled outside to make a phone call and noticed the memorial he and Jesse had built for the September 11 dead. Wanting to get a better view of the shrine, he crossed the street, lit a cigarette, and sat down on the train tracks to reflect.

That's the last thing Cameron remembers before a freight train ran him over.

Others tell him that the train cut off his legs first, way up high above his knees. Then the impact flipped his body over and his right arm got caught under the train. The engineer of the freight train called 911, and miraculously, Cameron survived long enough for the paramedics to put tourniquets on his severed limbs. They put his legs on ice, but there was nothing left to his arm—only a hand.

The doctors in the emergency room didn't expect him to live. His family was called to come say good-bye, but Jesse was nowhere to be found. He had run away after hearing the sirens, knowing something horrible had happened the way only an identical twin can.

The next thing Cameron remembered was waking up in the ICU three days later, sensing that something was very, very wrong.

When he opened his eyes, his whole family was there, and the first thing he felt was an overwhelming feeling of gratitude.

His first words were to his father. "Hey, did we find that bastard Osama bin Laden yet?"

Then Cameron looked down to see that his legs weren't there. He looked to his right side and saw that his right arm was gone too. In a panic, he looked down between the stumps of his legs to see if what he called his "manhood" was still there. He breathed a sigh of relief to discover that it was. At least he had that, he thought.

After three weeks of rapid progress in the hospital, when Cameron was finally discharged, that's when the fear and grief that had mostly spared him in the hospital swept over him. Wanting to avoid the pain of facing all he had lost, Cameron went back to partying, which was particularly hard on his family. They had to witness Cameron's transformation from the handsome, active, confident, independent, funny teenager to a disabled, depressed, insecure, sedentary, substance-abusing teenager who needed help doing anything.

Cameron was on a downward spiral for seven years. Then one day in 2008, he discovered that his twin Jesse's room was locked. Cameron and Jesse were living together, and Cameron got a bad feeling about the locked door, so he busted it down with his prosthetic leg and found his twin lying on his bed, dead from an overdose. Cameron says it was the worst day of his life.

Right after Jesse's death, Cameron got very sick with a high fever, and he called 911. While he was recovering from an infection, Cameron realized he was at a critical choice point. He could let Jesse's death be the last straw in a life that was going down the tubes. Or he could tap into an inner strength he barely knew even existed within him. Cameron chose life.

When I asked Cameron what helped him make that choice, he said, "I had people I could count on. I had a girlfriend who helped me a lot at the time, even though we had broken up. My spiritual life also got me through, my belief in a power greater than myself. I read Eckhart Tolle's *The Power of Now* and *A New Earth*. That was a springboard for my spiritual growth, my self-esteem, and my confidence. That was my turnaround. My brother lost his life. I almost lost mine. But life is too precious. We're lucky to get a chance to make our lives mean something. I had to grow up and take responsibility for the rest of my life."

After that wake-up call, Cameron had to deal with his anger and grief, then buckle down—literally: to strap on his prosthetic legs and get back to life. This required adjusting his attitude, visualizing where he wanted to be, making a plan, and committing to radical change.

After becoming self-sufficient with two prosthetic legs and a prosthetic arm, Cameron was able to get a job working as a patient advocate and speaking at workshops held by physical and occupational therapists. Soon afterward, he was asked to give his first big inspirational speech at an inner-city high school in Minneapolis on Valentine's Day.

A few days later, he got an e-mail from a foster child girl who didn't feel loved by anyone—not her foster parents, not her friends, and not by the boyfriend she didn't have. She said she went home after Cameron's speech, and although she had been contemplating suicide, she flushed all the pills down the toilet and decided she was going to take action. She had a heart-to-heart with her foster parents, talked to her counselor at school about how she was being bullied, and decided to choose life like Cameron had.

This defining moment made Cameron realize that he had a real opportunity to serve others. He tried to make his message his brother's legacy. Since then, he has learned to run, surf, ski, and golf on his prostheses, and he now serves as a camp counselor at Camp No Limits, helping young kids with limb loss learn to make the most out of life. He also participates in Operation Surf, a surf clinic for injured service member amputees. He said, "I go out there as an ambassador. I paddle out there with these short feet called 'stubbies' and surf waves with these guys."

Cameron could have chosen to let his life be ruled by fear, but instead, he chose to let his greatest fears heal him. When you let loss initiate you rather than destroy you, when you allow life to be your teacher, even the most tragic loss can be a blessing. Cameron probably once believed in Fearful Assumption #2:

"I can't handle losing what I cherish." And yet, after the tragic losses he has experienced at such a young age, I suspect he might now embrace Courage-Cultivating Truth #2: "Loss is natural and can lead to growth." Having demonstrated not only that he can handle what most people would consider their worst nightmare, but also that he can alchemize loss into an opportunity to realize his life's purpose, Cameron can help us identify times in our own lives when we experience that loss is natural and can lead to growth.

FEAR AND VULNERABILITY

If we're willing to let them, pain, grief, and loss are here to wake us up from the mindless slumber of the Small Self and free us from the soul cage of false fear. Graciously receiving such a gift does not come easily to most of us. In modern culture, we tend to have an unhealthy relationship with loss. In indigenous cultures, loss is more easily accepted as a natural part of life. But in our materialistic modern culture, we have no cultural mythology that helps us deal with loss, so we become loss averse. We view loss as failure, rather than being willing to accept it or even embrace it for the teachings that accompany it. We punish children by taking things away from them. We reward them by giving them things. We train our children to associate loss with personal failure, shame, guilt, and being "bad." Loss is not seen as a natural part of life and welcomed as an essential part of growth. Instead, we resist loss at all costs, which means we also resist change, since change always requires loss in some form. Nothing begins without something ending.

In order to avoid change and its accompanying loss, we are willing to tolerate stagnation, to let our souls die slow deaths in order to avoid uncertainty and loss. Anything that requires risk becomes unacceptable. This is how fear is born. Dress rehearsing tragedy is just one way we armor against the vulnerability of love and loss, which triggers a feeling that Brené Brown calls "foreboding joy."

Most of us have experienced this: awash in gratitude for all we have, we are suddenly bulldozed by a fear of having it taken away.

In her research, Brené Brown was shocked to discover when people reported feeling their most vulnerable. Often, it's when things are going best for us—when we're standing over our children while they're sleeping, or loving our jobs, or going into remission, or falling in love.

In other words, we're most afraid when we feel we have the most to lose. Because we care *so much,* we love *so much,* we have *so much,* we are terrified that we might blink and lose it all. And the reality is, we might. Life is impermanent, and nothing we do can protect us against this harsh truth.

Because we can't tolerate this truth, we armor against it with a variety of tools Brené Brown calls "vulnerability armor." Foreboding joy is one type of armor. But there are others, like perfectionism. Perfectionism stems from fear, because we're afraid that if we fail to be perfect, we'll disappoint others, be rejected, fail, and be ostracized by those whose approval matters to us. Perfectionism is not the same as striving for excellence. It's the misguided belief that if we abide by some external definition of "perfect," we will be protected from the shame, blame, and judgment we most fear.

Numbing is another vulnerability shield. Because we're not well equipped to handle our fear of loss, shame, blame, and judgment, we numb out with alcohol, cigarettes, drugs, food, sex, caffeine, even my addiction of choice—busyness.

It's natural to try to armor ourselves from the vulnerability we feel when faced with the reality that every blessing holds within it the risk of loss. A healthier approach lies in learning to make peace with that vulnerability. But how do we do this? How do we comfort ourselves in a world that threatens to expose us to what we most fear or take away from us what we most cherish?

The vulnerability of how much you have to lose can gut you. You may find yourself closing your heart, even to those you love most, because you just can't bear the thought of losing what you cherish so much. Fear is born here too.

LOSS AS AN INITIATION

We hate to face this painful truth, but life is impermanent. Everything we cherish we will one day lose. And life most often teaches us our greatest lessons through the vehicle of loss. Loss, if we let it, can initiate us into a soul-driven life. Loss can lead to a sort of rebirth that matures us, grows the wisdom within us, and opens a door to the next phase of our growth.

In her book *Broken Open,* Elizabeth Lesser writes, "Adversity is a natural part of being human. It is the height of arrogance to prescribe a moral code or health regime or spiritual practice as an amulet to keep things from falling apart. Things do fall apart. It is in their nature to do so. When we try to protect ourselves from the inevitability of change, we are not listening to the soul. We are listening to our fear of life and death, our lack of faith, our smaller ego's will to prevail. To listen to the soul is to stop fighting with life—to stop fighting when things fall apart; when they don't go our way, when we get sick, when we are betrayed or mistreated or misunderstood. To listen to the soul is to slow down, to feel deeply, to see ourselves clearly, to surrender to discomfort and uncertainty, and to wait."

Whether the adversity we fear or have already faced is the death of a loved one, a divorce, the loss of a job, the dissolution of a romance, the loss of good health, or a financial loss, when we lose what we cherish, we have a choice. We can break down or we can break open, as Lesser describes. A breakdown in the wake of loss can lead to fear, depression, anxiety, isolation, addiction, or cynicism, and make us emotionally unavailable or unable to cope. It may even lead to illness or suicide. But there's another way to respond to loss. Loss can lead to an unexpected blossoming. Through it, we can become more of who we really are than we ever thought possible.

Many of us walk around surrounded by a shell that protects us from the outside world. Whether we like it or not, loss offers the opportunity to crack the shell. Having your shell cracked in the wake of loss can feel unbearably painful; you may feel like a raw neuron, unprotected from everything that threatens to prick you, and want to put on even stronger armor. But this isn't the only way to deal with loss. You can choose to let it break you open and leave you that way, available for living a richer, deeper life with your heart wide open.

How we deal with adversity affects how courageous we can become. Whether we're talking about illness, the loss of a loved one, heartbreak, career disappointment, financial problems, or sexual abuse, it's so easy to fall into victim mode and feel helpless, at the mercy of what feels like a hostile universe. We may not be able to change the circumstance of what happens, but we can always put on new lenses and view the adversity with a new perspective.

What if, instead of being victims of adversity, our souls—on some level—choose these challenges as a way to help us grow? I once gently asked someone with Stage 4 cancer whether she thought it was possible that her soul and God sat down for tea before she was ever born and decided that, in order for her to grow into the enlightened being she was becoming, she would need to get cancer at a young age. Is it possible that cancer or abuse or divorce or bankruptcy might be *necessary* for spiritual development?

Back in 2006, when my Perfect Storm blew through, I felt like a victim of a hostile universe, and I thought I would never survive the pummeling of adversity. But now, through the lens of my "retrospectoscope," I see that it was all perfectly orchestrated to crack the shell of my ego and spawn me toward who I was meant to become. My soul chose well, even though my Small Self hated it all. I can now say that my Perfect Storm is the best thing that ever happened to me, because it woke me up from my unconsciousness.

We can all try to remember this whenever things don't go the way our Small Selves wish they would. Whenever adversity strikes, first we need to grieve and feel our genuine emotions, but then we can choose to put on different lenses. "Look! Soul growth! Bring it on. Let's lean in and milk it for all it's worth."

When adversity strikes, it's so tempting to attach to the outcome we want. Whenever I find myself praying for what I want, I remind myself of a Taoist story I love.

An old farmer had been tending his crops for many years when his horse ran away. When his neighbors heard the news, they sympathized. "Such bad luck."

The farmer said, "Maybe."

The next morning, the horse appeared, bringing with it three other wild horses. The neighbors said, "How wonderful! Lucky you!"

"Maybe," replied the old man.

The following day, the farmer's son hopped on the back of one of the untamed horses, but the horse bucked him off, and he broke his leg. The neighbors said, "How tragic. Such misfortune."

"Maybe," answered the farmer.

The next day, military officials arrived in the village to draft young men into the army. When they came across the old farmer's son and saw his injury, they passed him by. The neighbors congratulated the farmer on how well things had turned out.

"Maybe," said the farmer.

When adversity strikes, we just never know when something that looks like misfortune may actually be a blessing. So I've stopped praying for what I want. Instead, I simply offer up this prayer: "May the highest come into being."

ENDBEGINNINGS

When Rachel Naomi Remen and I were sitting at her kitchen table, talking about a healthy way to view loss, she told me this story from her book *Kitchen Table Wisdom*:

I was 35 years old before I understood that there is no ending without a beginning. That beginnings and endings are always right up against each other.

That was the year I first went to Esalen Institute. I was just learning how to make jewelry and had cast a silver ring. I was proud of the design. At that time many craftsman were in residence at Esalen and the ring attracted a great deal of admiration and attention. Several suggested that I drive back up the coast a few miles and show it to the jeweler at a gallery we had passed on the road.

It was about to rain, but I made the trip anyway. The jeweler loved the design, and I left my ring with him so that he could recast it and sell it to others. I drove back down Route 1 to Esalen with difficulty. Some serious rain had begun.

During the night, a wild and violent storm hit the coast. At breakfast I was shocked to hear that we were isolated. A two-mile stretch of Route 1 just north of Esalen had fallen into the ocean. The gallery was gone and my ring with it. Through my numbness, I could hear several inner voices commenting on my loss. The loudest was my father's saying, "This never would have happened if you hadn't allowed a total stranger to exploit you." And my mother's: "You can never be trusted with anything valuable." Mixed in was the voice of a very young part of myself that kept looking at the place on my hand where the ring had been yesterday and saying, "Where is it? It was right here."

In anguish, I went to the edge of the cliffs and stood looking down at the Pacific, still wild from yesterday's storm. Down there somewhere was my ring. As I watched the ocean hammer the cliffs, it began to occur to me that there was something natural, even inevitable, about what had happened. Pieces of the United States had been falling into the ocean for thousands of years. Perhaps all those familiar blaming voices were wrong. There was nothing at all personal in it, just some larger process at work.

I looked at the place on my finger again. This time it really was an empty space. For the first time I faced a loss with a sense of curiosity. What would come to fill up this space? Would I make another ring? Or find one in a thrift shop or a foreign country? Or would someone give me a ring someday because he loved me?

I was 35 years old and I had never trusted life before. Anything I had ever let go of had claw marks on it. But this empty space was different.

PERMISSION TO BREAK YOUR HEART

Letting go of precious objects, money that supports a certain lifestyle, social status, or professional kudos can be exceptionally painful, especially if we've wrapped our value around such things. This kind of loss triggers primal survival instincts, which often revolve around childhood traumas that surface in the face of loss in order to be healed. Letting go in relationships may be the trickiest of all losses, because such loss elicits feelings of rejection, abandonment, insecurity, and unworthiness, which also tend to stem from childhood wounds.

Somehow, I inherited a belief that all relationships, especially those with people I love deeply, are meant to last forever. I always figured that if I love someone, we should both be sitting next to each other in our rocking chairs when we're 90, and if we're not, it's because somebody screwed up, probably me. My therapist jokes that I'm a doctor, so it's in my nature to do CPR on dead things. I have a tendency to go overboard to try to save a relationship I value, even when it's obvious to everyone else that it's over. But someone once told me people come into our lives for a reason, a season, or a lifetime. Knowing how to discern the difference is a skill worth acquiring.

It's part of the human condition to suffer from the broken heart. Every single one of us has experienced this trauma at some point in our lives. The pain can feel so unbearable that we armor up against it, often shutting out intimacy before it even happens. My daughter, Siena, and I have discussed this often. When Siena was five, her heart got broken by a little girl named Vivien, the daughter of my best friend, born two weeks after Siena. Siena and Vivien had known each other since they were three months old, but they hadn't actually seen each other since, because Siena and I lived in San Francisco and Vivien lived in Chicago. Siena had heard great tales of Princess Vivien, and Vivien had heard wondrous stories of Siena and her fairy magic. But finally, they were together in one place when my best friend and Vivien came to visit. They got to chase fairies in a Zen garden, play on the beach, sleep in the same bed every night, bathe together with Roberto the toy penguin, eat fish and chips at the English pub, watch fireworks over San Francisco on the 4th of July, listen to a dharma talk about *Harold and the Purple Crayon* at Green Gulch Zen Center, spend hours in a hot tub, and share other magical adventures that made them fall in love. They were so in love that Siena pretty much ignored me, her father, and my visiting best friend that entire week.

But then life as the teacher showed up, and Vivien had to go back home to Chicago.

Siena wept when she left. Inconsolably. For hours. She threw herself onto her bed and pointed to the trundle bed where Vivien had slept and said, "Every time I look at her bed and she's not there, my heart hurts." Then she wept some more. A friend of mine had just died, so I cried when she said this, because my heart hurt too.

Siena said, "Mommy, it hurts so much to love Vivien that I don't think I ever want to see her again."

That's when I realized we needed to have a talk. I curled Siena up on my lap and told her I understood how much it hurts when someone you love has to go. I assured her it was all worth it. I told her that the loving is worth the leaving and that in order to fully experience the joy of loving others, we have to be willing to lose them. I said, "We have to give those we love permission to break our hearts."

She looked at me with a furrowed brow and said, "But Mommy, I would never, ever break your heart."

I said, "Ah, but you might. Without even meaning to. You could leave me, and I would cry, and I would look at your bed, and I might wish you had never slept in it because it would hurt so much that you're not there."

Siena started to cry and said, "But I would never do that to you, Mommy. I would never leave you. I will always love you and live in this house with you until I'm old."

I told her how I had given my father—her Papa—permission to break my heart—and when he died two weeks after she was born during my Perfect Storm, he did. He cracked it *wide open* and it spilled all over the floor and made me think about sewing it shut with big wire sutures that would keep it closed forever. But then I decided to keep my heart open, in spite of how much it hurt. I told Siena that someday, someone she loved, someone she gave permission to break her heart—like me or her father or her Nana or our dog, Grendel—might break her heart, and she might feel just like she did at that moment, like she didn't want to give anyone permission to do that ever again. She might want to shut down her heart so it wouldn't hurt like it did when Vivien left.

Siena got it. She said, "Mama, when you fall in love, you should always leave a little crack in your heart, even when you feel like you should lock it. And that way, the right person can always sneak in."

I nodded, and we cried some more. Then I held her for a long time.

Right before she fell asleep, Siena said, "I'm going to give Princess Vivien permission to break my heart."

I said, "I think that's a good plan." We spun the dream catcher, and turned the lights out.

A year later, when Siena was six, our beloved Grendel died quickly and unexpectedly of sudden heart failure, and the grief felt almost unbearable. As we held Grendel's dead body in our arms, Siena wailed like we all wanted to and said, "Grendel, I gave you permission to break my heart, and you went and broke it." We were at the veterinary hospital, and even the staff wept.

Two months after we lost Grendel, when our hearts were still raw from the loss, Siena said, "Mama, I'm ready to give another dog permission to break my heart." We talked about how dogs don't live as long as humans and how getting another dog meant we would likely have to endure the same kind of loss one day. But, I reassured her, we could hope that a new puppy would live at least ten years before we had to say good-bye again. Siena nodded her agreement, and two-month-old Bezoar joined our family.

Six months later, I could barely breathe when I got the phone call from the kind man calling from Highway 1, tearfully confessing that he had just run over Bezoar in his car. Siena and I buried her tiny body next to Grendel.

It has taken us a while to recover from the back-to-back losses, but Siena came to me recently and said, "Mama, I'm ready again. I'm ready to let another dog break my heart." Soon, we will once again invite another dog into our lives, and we will love fiercely until it breaks us open yet again.

We've all had our hearts broken, over and over. The hardest thing you'll ever do is keep your heart open in the face of serial heartbreak. Closing off your heart is the easy way out. It makes sense. Nobody would blame you. But then you'd miss out on the love.

Life is full of traumas to the heart, and perhaps more than anything else, it triggers false fear because we're so afraid of heartbreak. Love feels risky. Love feels unsafe. Love feels like something to protect against. But closing the heart is never the solution.

TODAY IS A GOOD DAY TO DIE

It's impossible to consider our discomfort with the unknown without pointing out the elephant in the room—*death*. Not only our pets', but our own. Most people perceive death as the ultimate loss, though perhaps it is the ultimate beginning. We can't really know what happens beyond death, because death is a mystery. Every religious tradition has its own beliefs about what lies beyond death, but when it comes right down to it, science can't prove what comes next. We can only be curious. Is life over once our hearts stop beating? Is there a heaven? Does hell exist? Is there a long-bearded God who sits in judgment and decides where we go? Do we reincarnate into other human bodies? Do we become angels? Do we become ghostly spirits, sticking around the earthly plane to haunt humans? Do we come back in some other form? Or do we simply decompose in soil-filled graves and cease to exist? The truth is that *nobody knows for sure,* and this fills us with fear.

What if we could know? What if we knew with certainty that death was nothing to fear? What if we weren't afraid to lose our own lives or those we love because we knew that what came next was actually an upgrade? What if death represented not failure or loss, but the natural course of the soul's journey once it has learned what it's here in human form to learn? As we discussed in Chapter 2, imagine how things might be different if health care professionals didn't fear death. How might health care change if we trusted death as a natural, even welcome part of life? Would we stop grasping at every little test and treatment that might prolong life? How might end-of-life care change?

How might a peaceful acceptance of the inevitability of death affect all our other fears? Perhaps we wouldn't be so afraid of suicide bombers or the Ebola virus or plane crashes. We might stop living in fear of pesticides in our food and nuclear bombs and hurricanes. We live in a world filled with uncertainty, but if we weren't afraid to die or lose someone we loved, perhaps we'd be less ruled by our fears. And how would that feel? What would life be like if we were less afraid?

Because so many of us have such an unhealthy relationship with death, we forget that death is a natural part of life. As Marilyn Schlitz, Ph.D., and Deepak Chopra, M.D., say in their documentary film by the same name, "Death makes life possible." Only through a healthy relationship with the inevitability of death will we come into right relationship with our fear of loss. This is not to suggest that we shouldn't try to avoid death when we can. No need to tumble over a cliff if we can simply step back from the edge. Sure, it's not a bad idea to avoid walking around dark alleys in dangerous neighborhoods at midnight. It's worth teaching our children not to jump into swimming pools when they don't know how to swim. There's nothing wrong with surgery, chemotherapy, and radiation when facing a cancer diagnosis. This is why true fear can increase the length of time we're blessed to live. But assuming that we're mindful about doing what's within our power to enjoy a long, healthy life, perhaps we can see death as a natural part of life, not something to fear but the beginning of what's next.

Whenever I think about death, I can't help thinking about Lee Lipsenthal, M.D., a physician who spent much of his career working with Dean Ornish, M.D., and teaching physicians how to find balance in a medical life. Lee lived by the credo "Today is a good day to die." Lee didn't have a death wish. His friends and students knew what he meant—that every day, every bit of love had been expressed, that every dream had been fulfilled, that Lee didn't hold back from living the richest expression of life that he could, and that death is nothing to fear when you have no regrets. Such a philosophy is easier said than done when you've just been given a terminal cancer diagnosis at a young age, as Lee was. In his book *Enjoy Every Sandwich,* Lee wrote, "I . . . knew that the more fear and anxiety I had, the higher my stress hormone levels would be. High stress hormones wear down the immune system's function over time, giving cancer a better chance to grow. Fear promotes cancer growth; calm decreases it. My mode of being became 'get quiet, enjoy life, and let my body do what it knows how to do—cure cancer.'"

In the end, cancer won, but until then, Lee enjoyed every sandwich—BLTs, to be specific. If we're willing to face it, the inevitability of death grants us the opportunity to relish the blessing of life while we still have it.

THE GAME OF LIFE

Some teachers and researchers, such as psychologist Michael Newton, Ph.D., who examined the experience of his patients under hypnosis, posit that life on earth is in essence a school for the soul: here, we live out the challenges and triumphs and, yes, losses we have chosen in order to learn and grow. I'm not suggesting we should skip straight from grief to gratitude when we lose what we cherish. Don't even think about telling a grieving parent who has just lost a child, "Don't worry, his soul and yours agreed that he would die young so you could learn the spiritual lesson of nonattachment." This is not helpful when someone is in the throes of human grief.

Knowing that loss can initiate you and trusting that every struggle comes hand in glove with soul growth doesn't diminish the pain of loss when you're in the heartbreak of it all. But when you look back, you may start to see the gifts. Over time, once you've experienced enough loss, you'll start to sense the growth opportunities in such moments, and the knowledge that growth accompanies loss can help ease the suffering.

To get this perspective, I find it helpful to practice observing my life from the witness position. Martha Beck makes the analogy of playing a video game. As a human, you can get very engaged in one of these games. Some of them are so real that you start to fully identify with your video game avatar. Your avatar may have a name, a costume, a personality, and special skills that equip you to play your best. You may get so lost in the game that you forget to eat or pee or feed your kids. You might be so engrossed that if someone were to interrupt you while you were playing the game, you'd startle, having briefly forgotten you're not your avatar. In truth, you're the human holding the joystick.

Now step back one more level. What if, instead of just being a human playing a video game, you're a soul playing a human who is playing a video game? What if your whole human life is as much of a game as the video game is? And what if you can manipulate the game of life, just as you manipulate the joystick? What if life is not some random, chaotic sequence of events, but a carefully orchestrated symphony of perfectly timed, artfully composed movements, conjured up between you and the spiritual forces that guide you to help you grow as a soul?

Think of the greatest challenges you've ever faced—childhood abuse, the abandonment or neglect of a parent, illness or disability, the loss of a loved one, betrayal, heartbreak, divorce, poverty, being the victim of a violent crime, selling your soul for a paycheck, or whatever has hurt you the most. What if, instead of being a victim of these traumas, on some soul level, you chose these challenges? This doesn't mean you condone wrongs perpetrated on you. It doesn't mean you don't deserve to be angry or grieving or heartbroken. But you can distance yourself enough from the game to see that there's a part of you that is safe from all this hurt, a part that is standing back, watching you feel what you feel and learn what you need to learn.

For us as humans, joy is fun. It's easeful. It's sexy and silly and hilarious and connecting. It's full of love and beauty and massages and heart-openings. Joy can teach us just as well as loss can. But joy tends to take longer, while loss puts us on the fast track.

Once you start viewing loss as an opportunity for growth and initiation, you stop fearing loss, you start accepting what is, and you absorb the lessons life on earth is trying to teach you. And once this happens, once you let yourself become a student of life, humbled by life, no longer resisting it, something shifts, and life no longer needs to teach you by whacking you with cosmic two-by-fours. Once one of your greatest fears comes true, you learn that you are not in control the way you thought you were, and you let go if you're willing to let fear cure you of your constant grasping. Once you learn what you're meant to learn from loss, you can lean into joy without holding back. Perhaps our ability to surrender into loss with an open heart is the measure of a successful life.

COURAGE-CULTIVATING EXERCISE #6

Be the Witness

When you find yourself getting mired in the emotions of loss (or any other painful emotions, for that matter), try this exercise, which helps you remember that you are not the avatar, getting shot at by life; you are the soul playing the video game of earth school.

If loss is causing you to suffer, notice the emotions you feel—grief, loneliness, anger, hurt, sadness, disappointment, anxiety, resentment. It's easy to mistakenly identify with those emotions as *who you are.* But what if instead of *being* the emotion, you are simply the soul who is *with* that emotion? What if, instead of saying "I am sad," you shift to "I am *with* sad"? What if, instead of being a sad person, you are the expanse of consciousness witnessing the part of you that feels sad?

Try the following exercise:

1. If you start to feel an emotional disturbance, such as anger, frustration, sadness, or hurt, name the feeling and notice it.

2. Step back and witness the part of you that is disturbed by this feeling. You are not this feeling. The part of you that is feeling this feeling is your avatar. You are the soul who is witnessing the angry, hurting avatar.

3. Close your eyes and give yourself as much time as you need to fully witness the emotional disturbance. Let your soul offer love, compassion, and comfort to the avatar part of you that is suffering.

Even in the midst of negative emotions, the expanse of pure consciousness that is *you* at the soul level can be at peace, even when the avatar part of you is grieving or hurt or angry. You can ride the emotions like a wave, and they will pass right through you. Studies show that most emotions last no longer than 90 seconds unless we attach stories to them. You have a feeling of being lonely—and this will pass through you quickly unless you make up a story about how you're lonely because you're unlovable and worthless and nobody will *ever* love you and you're going to be alone forever. When you attach to the story, you suffer needlessly and the suffering can linger for years. But you don't have to choose to suffer this way. Your soul can find peace, comfort, and stillness even in the most difficult times if you're able to view your negative emotions from this witness position.

COURAGE-CULTIVATING EXERCISE #7

"I Accept" Meditation

Most of the unnecessary pain we experience when we face loss stems from our resistance to the loss. Because we falsely assume that whatever we once had should last forever, we resist, yet the resistance causes more suffering than the loss itself. Next time you find yourself resisting loss, try closing your eyes and spending 20 minutes in meditation repeating the mantra, "I accept." When you accept what is rather than resisting, you come closer to freeing yourself from unnecessary suffering.

This sounds easier than it is. It's no small feat to accept cancer, the death of a child, the loss of a limb, getting fired, the end of a romance, or bankruptcy. But resisting won't bring back what you've lost. If you find this exercise challenging, go back to Courage-Cultivating Exercise #6 and practice being the witness. Notice the part of you that resists your loss, and open your heart with compassion to your avatar self that doesn't want to accept what is. Love and accept even that part of you. Acceptance is your key to freedom.

To listen to a free "I Accept" meditation, download the free Prescription for Courage kit at TheFearCureBook.com.

Courage-Cultivating Exercise #8

Find Gratitude in Loss

Pull out your journal and reflect on a loss in your life. Maybe a loved one died, or maybe you were abandoned by a parent or rejected by a lover. Maybe you lost your money or your house or your pet or your best friend. Maybe you had to let go of a dream or say good-bye to perfect health. Don't ignore any sad, hurt, or angry feelings that come up, but do allow yourself to shift your focus so you can pay attention to any blessings that may have arisen as a result of the loss. Have you ever felt that a loss is initiating you into some new phase of life? Has your heart opened? Has your soul grown because of what you experienced? Write down your reflections.

CHAPTER 6

IT'S *a* PURPOSEFUL UNIVERSE

The most important decision we make is whether we
believe we live in a friendly or hostile universe.

— ALBERT EINSTEIN

Since she was a child, Trish had always been terrified of snakes. When she was little, her family vacationed at a place with an outhouse, and she had always been warned that snakes can live in the outhouse toilets, where they can lurk in the dark before jumping up and biting you when you're sitting on the pot. Because of this, she was always on the lookout for snakes in toilets.

She never saw a snake in the outhouse toilet when she was a child, but as an adult, all snakes, even harmless little garter snakes, left her quaking in her sneakers. One night, Trish and her husband were at the farmhouse they owned on 40 acres of rustic countryside in the North Georgia mountains when she had to go to the bathroom. She looked in the toilet first, as she always did, and then sat down and peed. When she was done, she stood up, and seeing something brown in the toilet when she hadn't moved her bowels, she did a double take.

That's when her husband heard her let out a bloodcurdling scream.

There, in the bowl of the toilet, was a large poisonous cottonmouth snake, swimming happily in the water. She hadn't seen it when she first went to sit down. It must have been hidden under the rim of the wooden toilet seat. With no easy way to remove the snake from the toilet until they could get help in the morning, Trish was terrified to stay in the farmhouse that night. She insisted upon leaving the house until her husband found a way to block the bathroom door, trapping the snake in the bathroom if it somehow escaped the toilet bowl.

The next morning, the snake was not visible in the toilet any longer, so Trish's husband called a plumber, who showed up, ironically, with a "plumber's snake," meant to get rid of anything that might be blocking the drain pipes. Unfortunately, when the plumber "snaked" the pipes, the cottonmouth was killed. The plumber removed pieces of it until the pipes were clear, thinking Trish's fears would be relieved after that.

But the nightmare wasn't over. In the course of the next day, Trish found 13 baby cottonmouths all over the house—in a teapot, on the staircase, under a carpet, under a pile of clothes. Perhaps the mama cottonmouth had come inside to lay eggs. Maybe the babies were coming out of the sinks through the pipes. It was hard to say how they got there.

Trish never could relax in that farmhouse after that. It's been empty now for years, but she's still afraid to go back and get the house ready to sell. Her husband died years ago and she can't face going back alone. And she still has to psych herself up every time she gets near a toilet, reminding herself that what happened is in the past and that there's not likely to be a real snake under the toilet seat ever again.

What Trish experienced when she saw that cottonmouth in her toilet was true fear. She really could have been hurt by that poisonous snake, so her initial reaction was appropriate. But the snake phobia that has shadowed her since is understandable false fear. When you experience something terrifying and life-threatening like this, it's easy to conclude that you live in a dangerous world, and the conclusion gets reinforced by your neurobiology. Trish's amygdala, which helps form "implicit memories," stored this snake experience deep in her unconscious mind, and as her limbic brain kept getting repetitively triggered, the amygdala tinged these memories with more and more fear residues. When this happens, fear takes on a life of its own, and it's easy to conclude that the world must be a dangerous place where we always need to be on the alert.

Originally, Trish's stress responses were triggered by a real threat (true fear). Poisonous snakes in your house are a danger in need of a remedy. But once the snakes were gone, what remained—fear of toilets and an even more generalized undercurrent of chronic fear—was a remembered or imagined threat (false fear). This is a warning system malfunction, alerting us to dangers that don't actually threaten us. And it's really nothing but a thought—*I live in a dangerous world.*

If we question Fearful Assumption #3, "It's a dangerous world," we could probably brainstorm lots of counterarguments providing evidence to contradict this thought. As Albert Einstein said, "The most important decision we make is whether we believe we live in a friendly or hostile universe." Because Trish is my mother, I know she has collected mounds of evidence that it's not really a dangerous world, in spite of what happened with the snakes. Mom is a woman of great faith, so she used the power of her mighty mind to round up all the evidence she could that she lives in a friendly universe. She has witnessed what felt like very purposeful miracles. She has witnessed encounters with what she considers angels. She feels the intimate presence of a divine force in her life. And she trusts that when things happen that her Small Self doesn't want, they're happening for a purpose.

Mom's two biggest fears were living alone and snakes. First she survived the snake incident, and then my father died during my Perfect Storm, leaving her alone for the last nine years. Sitting with me on the dock on the lake by her house where she used to live with my father, she said, "Maybe this all happened so I could learn that even if what I fear most happens, I can handle it. Once I've survived that, I guess I can handle anything."

When I asked Mom whether she believed it was possible that her biggest fears came true for some cosmic purpose so she could grow, she conceded that this might be possible. Could she buy into the idea that it's a purposeful universe?

Mom nodded.

LIFE IN A "DANGEROUS WORLD"

Do we live in a dangerous world? After the events of September 11, many people certainly thought so. In the wake of that tragedy, people were so afraid of being killed in a plane hijacking that many switched from flying to driving, even though the biggest risk of traveling by plane is the drive to the airport. In fact, one professor calculated that even if terrorists were hijacking and crashing one jet per week, a person flying once a month would only have a 1-in-135,000 chance of being killed in a plane hijacking, a miniscule risk compared to the annual 1-in-6,000 risk of being killed in a car crash.

In fact, Gerd Gigerenzer, a Berlin psychologist, anticipating that September 11 would lead to more traffic fatalities that year, began tracking the data. As expected, fatalities on American roads soared after September 11. Gigerenzer was able to ferret out the number of unnecessary car crash fatalities that happened only because people were now more afraid of flying. The number was 1,595—more than half the number of those who died in the terrorist attacks. Irrational fear caused 1,595 people to die unnecessarily.[1]

The fear that paralyzed the nation didn't stop at fear of plane travel. When anthrax infected 22 people through the mail in the fall of 2001, 30,000 people began taking the antibiotic Cipro, often without a prescription. More people likely got sick from this powerful and dangerous superdrug than the 22 people who were infected with anthrax. Fear didn't protect them. It put them at further risk.

Then the nation experienced more health scares. In 2002, news broke that some of the smallpox virus stockpiled in the former Soviet Union might have found its way into the hands of terrorists. Smallpox fears escalated, even though there hasn't been a case of smallpox in the United States since the 1940s. In 2003, when severe acute respiratory syndrome (SARS) emerged in Asia, there were only 7,000 cases in the entire world and less than 100 in the United States. But that didn't keep Americans from wearing masks, boycotting plane travel, and avoiding Chinese restaurants.

When news of swine flu hit the media in 2009, hundreds of thousands of people began stockpiling the antiviral Tamiflu, while rushing to hospitals for even the slightest symptom. In 2011, when an earthquake caused a tsunami to devastate the Fukushima nuclear power plant in Japan, people as far away as the United States began buying up the nation's supply of potassium iodide, believed to help protect the thyroid gland from radiation exposure, until prices of the limited supply of the supplement began skyrocketing on eBay.

The public's wildly overblown reaction to these health scares—which in the big picture of the world's woes posed minimal risk—highlights something tragic happening in the modern psyche. We're not just afraid of real threats to our lives, the ones true fear can serve to protect us from. We're also afraid of rare, usually nonfatal viruses and far off, undetectable levels of radiation.

Yes, there are real dangers in our world, but we've lost touch with the statistical likelihood of these dangers, and as a result, many of us live in chronic fear. We're afraid of pesticides, hormones in milk, chemicals in food, poisons in our water supply, genetically modified organisms, and toxins in our air. We're worried about mercury in our fish and fillings, bacteria in our cheese, lead in our paint, leaky breast implants, and mold in our basements. We're afraid of toxins in our cosmetics, poisons in plastics, and contamination of our meat. We're anxious about whether microwave ovens, cell phones, and deodorant will kill us. We're terrified of cancer, AIDS, Alzheimer's, and herpes.

As if that's not enough, we also fear pedophiles, terrorists, shark attacks, methamphetamine, car accidents, tornados, and pit bulls. We've been afraid of global warming, nuclear war, Y2K, meteors, extraterrestrials, the end of the Mayan calendar, and "the big one" striking a major city. We're frightened of school shootings, movie theater shootings, drive-by shootings, and car bombs. We fear for our safety on a daily basis and wonder whether we'll ever again feel like we're out of harm's way.

And yet, in all measurable ways, we've never been safer. It's true across the developed world. Just for example, Americans enjoyed life spans 60 percent longer in 2000 than in 1900.[2] In 1900, a baby born in England had a life expectancy of 46 years. In 1980, it was 74 years. Today, in Canada, for example, the life expectancy is more than 80 years.

For most of human history, giving birth was the riskiest thing a woman could do. It still is for some women in developing countries, where 440 women die giving birth for every 100,000 children delivered. But in the developed world, only 20 out of 100,000 women die as a result of pregnancy. It's never been safer to have a baby.

Children are also safer than ever now. In England in 1900, 14 percent of all children died. By 1997, that number had fallen to 0.58 percent. While most parents confess to being terrified that they will lose a child, since 1970 alone, the death rate of American children has fallen by more than two-thirds.

We're not just living longer—we're living healthier. Fewer people develop chronic illnesses, and those who do get sick develop illnesses 10 to 25 years later in life than in years gone by. Even when people do get sick, the illnesses tend to be less severe. And people in developed countries today are less likely to become disabled.

We fear war, but from a historical perspective, we're living in one of the most peaceful times in human history. Fewer wars are being fought, and when war does happen, fewer people die. While people in developed countries are clearly more prosperous than those in developing countries, even those in developing countries are enjoying an improved quality of life. While still alarmingly high, the proportion of people in the developing world who are malnourished fell from 28 percent to 17 percent in the two decades following 1980.[3]

By all measures, we in the developed world are the healthiest, smartest, richest, safest people in human history. And yet, we have never been more afraid.

But it doesn't have to be this way . . .

IS IT A DANGEROUS WORLD?

When life has the potential to scare you with snakes in the toilet, cancers with no treatment, and genocide, it's no wonder people conclude that we live in a hostile universe. If you've suffered the traumas of abuse, abandonment, rejection, loss, illness, physical pain, the aftermath of violence, or other tragedies that leave you feeling unsafe, it's only natural to conclude that you live in a dangerous world. However, if you live on constant high alert, your body will get stuck in chronic repetitive stress response and you'll predispose your body to illness, in addition to making yourself needlessly unhappy.

Certainly, nobody is suggesting that the world doesn't hold real dangers. But is the thought "It's a dangerous world" true? What if you believed something different instead? What if, instead of a dangerous world, I suggest to you that it's a purposeful universe? Could you buy into that as an alternative?

When I suggest that we live in a purposeful universe rather than a dangerous world, I'm not suggesting that scary things don't happen or that you'll always be immune to tragedy. I'm not suggesting that you shouldn't be aware of danger or ignore all fear signals. I'm also not suggesting you'll always get what you want. What I am suggesting is that the universe may be orderly and meaningful even if we don't understand how it operates, and we may be protected by a loving Universal Intelligence that guides us through outer signs and inner knowing.

When you come to trust that you live in a purposeful rather than a hostile universe, false fear starts to lose its foothold. You develop a sense of safety that runs deeper than how much money is in your bank account or how much you feel loved by your spouse or whether or not your doctor gave you a clean bill of health. You begin to trust that whatever happens—even if it's not what you would have wished—contributes to your growth as a soul. When your commitment to soul growth supersedes your desire to get what you want, there's so much less to fear because you're not guarding against uncertainty or grasping at what you don't want to lose. This doesn't mean you don't take necessary steps to ensure your financial security, tend your relationships, guard against risk, or care for your body. It means you let go of the constant clutching for control.

Most of us are control freaks, and this attempt to control life leads to a lot of false fear. But when you believe you live in a purposeful universe, you realize the universe doesn't need you to be in charge, so you don't need to be afraid of letting go of the reins. Living in a purposeful universe allows you to come into right relationship with uncertainty because now, instead of viewing uncertainty with suspicion or fear, you can be at peace in the face of the unknown. Instead of guarding against loss, you can trust that even loss has a purpose, even if you don't know exactly what it is.

Once you begin to trust in this way, you'll find that false fear, while it may still show up, no longer rules your life. Instead of panicking when you lose your job, you trust that the perfect job will appear in the perfect timing. Instead of clinging to a love affair when it's ending, you trust that the dissolution of the relationship is a sign that a healthier, happier relationship is on the way. Instead of feeling afraid when you have a health scare, you have faith that whatever happens, it's all a welcome part of your soul's evolution. Even if you're faced with the ultimate bad news—that you may lose the life of a loved one or even your own life, you're able to trust the process and the outcome.

This doesn't mean you won't have emotional responses. If you lose a loved one, break up with someone you love, or face your own health battle, professional failure, or financial loss, of course you're going to experience grief, anger, and sadness. Trusting that you live in a purposeful universe is not about taking some spiritual bypass that skips you past painful emotions, but you don't have to get stuck in those emotions or in the victim stories that tend to arise when the universe doesn't deliver what you desired.

Living in a purposeful universe means that you have faith in a guiding force that is navigating life with you. You know that you are not alone, and this inner knowing offers protection against fear. The guiding force may organize around a religion you espouse as your own, or it may not. You may call this guiding force God or Buddha or Jesus or Allah or Quan Yin or the Divine or the Universe itself. You may perceive it as energy or even a wind of sorts, something that blows in the direction of the highest good and carries you with it if you let it. You may believe this guiding force comes from within you, or you may think of it as something outside of yourself.

It doesn't matter whether you believe this guidance comes from the deity of your choice, the Universe, energy, or your own Inner Pilot Light. What matters is that you trust that you don't have to micromanage every single little detail of your life because you know you are constantly being guided toward what is most aligned with the highest good, even if you don't know exactly what that will be. This guidance may be very subtle, but when you start to look for it, you'll see it more and more. Signs will guide your path. Synchronicities you can't explain will remind you that there is more than scientific materialism at work in the world around us. You may experience examples of extraordinary knowing, when you suddenly know something you shouldn't be able to know—something that helps you protect yourself or someone you know. You may even experience what seems like a miracle, and it may grant you the courage you thought you could never muster. This guiding force tends to pester you, and if you miss one sign, you're likely to receive another one.

15 Ways the Purposeful Universe Guides You

1. A persistent, seemingly irrational thought that won't go away

2. Dreams that offer you messages or suggestions

3. People who show up with messages for you at just the right time

4. Physical sensations or symptoms that arise from the body compass

5. Found objects that mean something to you

6. Inner voices and visions that arise during repetitive tasks, exercise, or meditation

7. Synchronicities that you might call coincidence, except that they feel too meaningful to be accidental

8. Books that speak directly to where you are in your life

9. Roadblocks that redirect you away from what you thought you wanted

10. Card decks, such as tarot or goddess cards

11. Animal totems that appear in your path

12. Song lyrics that you seem to hear over and over again

13. "Billboards" from the Universe, often in the form of license plates, bumper stickers, e-mails, or blog posts

14. Direct guidance offered by intuitive people

15. Numbers that have meaning to you, such as looking at the clock when it's 11:11

To learn how to notice and interpret the guidance that is always available to you, listen to 10 Ways Your Soul Guides You in Daily Life, a free teleclass with me and Rachel Naomi Remen, M.D. You can download the recording at no charge at MedicineForTheSoulRx.com.

"THIS CHANGES EVERYTHING"

Elizabeth Lloyd Mayer, Ph.D., author of *Extraordinary Knowing,* was a professor and researcher in the psychology department of the University of California at Berkeley and at the University Medical Center in San Francisco. Lisby, as she was known to her friends, was a skeptical scientist, not inclined to pay much attention to "woo woo" ideas. Then something unusual happened. In 1991, when her 11-year-old daughter Meg's handmade harp was stolen from the theater where she was playing, Lisby spent two months trying to recover the harp. The police got involved. She contacted instrument dealers all over the country. A CBS TV news story aired. But nothing worked. The harp was gone.

After she had given up hope, a friend of Lisby's said, "If you really want that harp back, you should be willing to try anything. What about calling a dowser?" Lisby had the kind of eyebrow-raising response most legitimate scientists would have to such a suggestion. From what she knew, dowsers were odd people who walked around with forked sticks telling you where to drill wells. But Lisby's friend told her that really good dowsers could find not just underground water, but also lost objects. Lisby didn't believe a dowser could find the harp, but with nothing to lose, she contacted the president of the American Society of Dowsers, Harold McCoy, in Fayetteville, Arkansas. She explained that a harp had been stolen from Oakland, California, and asked Harold if he could help her locate it.

Harold said, "Give me a second. I'll tell you if it's still in Oakland." He was silent for a moment and then said, "Well, it's still there. Send me a street map of Oakland and I'll locate that harp for you."

Lisby overnighted Harold a map of Oakland. Two days later, he called to give her the address where the harp was located. Lisby passed the information along to the police, who shook their heads. They couldn't issue a search warrant based on a hunch. So Lisby decided to drive to the address Harold had given her, where she posted flyers for two blocks around, offering a reward for the return of the harp.

Three days later, her phone rang. A man said that his neighbor had recently showed him the exact harp the flyer was describing. He said he would arrange to deliver it to her in the parking lot of an all-night Safeway. Lisby showed up at the appointed time and place, where a young man loaded the harp into the back of her station wagon.

Looking at the recovered harp, Lisby concluded, "This changes everything."

Lisby began asking colleagues and clients about their own "This changes everything" moments. What she discovered was that many people had had similar experiences of either personally knowing things they shouldn't have known or meeting someone who did in a way that felt extremely purposeful. She shared many of these stories of what scientists call "anomalous cognition" in *Extraordinary Knowing*. What I found most interesting about these stories of intuitive knowing was that what they knew didn't seem random. People weren't just intuiting what song was going to be on the radio next. Most of the time, what they extraordinarily knew contributed either to protecting themselves or to helping, comforting, or even saving the life of someone else.

One of the stories Lisby shared in *Extraordinary Knowing* was about a neurosurgeon who had been suffering from severe migraines that weren't responding to treatment. His doctor referred him for therapy with Lisby. Upon interviewing him, she discovered that his headaches had begun when he stopped teaching medical students and residents, which he loved. She asked why he had stopped teaching. He was reluctant to answer, but finally he confessed that he felt he couldn't explain to those he taught why he never seemed to lose a patient, in spite of the dangerous brain surgeries he performed. The reason, he finally explained, was that as soon as he realized his patient needed surgery, he camped out at the patient's bedside and waited . . . sometimes for 30 seconds, sometimes for hours. He waited for something he felt he couldn't explain to medical students or residents without them dismissing him as crazy. What he waited for was a distinctive white light that appeared around the patient's head. Until the light appeared, he knew it wasn't safe to operate. Once the light showed up, it was his signal to take the patient to the operating room: a purposeful sign, unexplainable by ordinary measures, that helped this doctor protect his patients.

Other psychologists and physicians shared similarly purposeful examples of extraordinary knowing with Lisby, often in hushed tones and under the promise of privacy. One of these distinguished psychoanalysts was Patrick Casement, whose books on clinical technique are considered psychology classics. He had heard about Lisby's experience with the harp and wanted to share his own story with her.

In 1952, when Casement was 17, he was staying with his father's mother for the Easter holidays. That week, his grandmother confided in him that she had only one real regret in her life. She had once deeply loved a dear friend, but during the war, when people kept relocating, the two of them lost touch. She had tried to find her friend, but all her efforts resulted in nothing more than returned letters.

On Easter Sunday, Casement attended a service at a church about four miles from his grandmother's house. Afterward, rather than taking the bus home, he decided to walk because he wanted to test out the solution he'd come up with to a school mathematics question. He had worked out exactly how fast he would have to walk so the bus couldn't catch up with him. He figured that if his calculations were wrong, he'd be able to hop on the bus and ride the rest of the way home. He was committed to walking those four miles at exactly the right pace, in order to prove that his mathematical calculations were correct.

But Casement's plan got derailed when, 20 minutes later, he surprised himself by sticking his thumb out to hitchhike. He said, "I was shocked to find that—in what I can only call a reflex action, as though my right arm had suddenly taken on a life of its own—I put out my right hand to thumb down one particular car. I was utterly astonished to watch myself defeating my own purpose. To my relief, the car drove past—my race against the bus was, I thought, not to be spoilt. But a moment later the car suddenly stopped. Since, regrettably, I had thumbed it down, I felt I had to accept the offered lift."

Casement got into the car and thanked the woman inside, who was being chauffeured by her driver. He imagined it must have been she who ordered the driver to go back and pick him up. The woman in the car asked Casement, "Were you at Winchester?" Casement had no idea what prompted the question, but he answered that yes, indeed, he was attending school at Winchester.

The woman in the car replied, "If you are there now, you won't know the person I am thinking of. He was called Roddie Casement and he went to Winchester, but that must have been a long time ago now." Roddie Casement was Patrick's father.

When he told her so, she was delighted. "Is his mother still alive?" she asked. Casement told her that not only was Roddie Casement's mother—Patrick's grandmother—still alive, but in fact, they would be driving right past her house two miles down the road. The lady then told Casement a story about how she had been trying to track down her very dear friend, whom she had lost touch with during the war. The friend she was seeking was Casement's grandmother, the same woman who had been searching for her. The two were reunited that day and spent the day together. Casement's grandmother died soon afterwards.

Reflecting back on what happened, Casement told Lisby, "Perhaps this lady saw a physical similarity between myself at seventeen and my father at a similar age. But that does not explain why my arm took on a life of its own and suddenly thumbed a lift from that particular car, forcing me to abandon my carefully calculated walk, the last thing I wanted to do. What I do know is accepting that lift meant my grandmother died happily, having finally met up with her beloved friend."

Maybe it was a coincidence, or maybe Casement's experience offers a bit of evidence of a purposeful universe. There's no way to prove it, but Lisby found that stories such as this one are common in the world of psychology and medicine.

Lisby spoke to one nurse who worked in the neonatal intensive care unit. This nurse often knew things she shouldn't have known, basing her clinical judgment on what she called "hunches." Her hunches saved a lot of babies' lives, and others on the unit came to trust them. Another doctor said to Lisby, "Because I'm so involved in getting to know [my patients], it's like I have a sense of smell—a literal *smell*—for how things are with them." She could smell death . . . literally. She could even smell where in the body disease was. She said, "It comes with a kind of certainty that is like smell, any smell that's strong and overpowering. You *know* you smell it, there's no doubt." This smell would guide her treatment decisions, but her boss would question her, and she didn't know how to rationalize her decisions. "What could I say—I got a *smell?*"

PURPOSE AND PROTECTION

What if the neurosurgeon really did see a white light around his patients' heads? What if this doctor really did get a smell? What if these doctors are being guided in some way in order to help save lives? Since Lisby had uncovered so many stories of health care providers who had intuitive experiences suggesting that we are being guided in some purposeful way, I thought I'd poke around and see if the people I knew had had any similar experiences.

My friend and mentor Rachel Naomi Remen, who was pediatric faculty at Stanford before writing *Kitchen Table Wisdom,* told me the story of a toddler who came into the emergency room at 3 A.M. one morning when she was a brand-new intern. The child seemed happy and lively, but his mother insisted he was in danger. "There is something terribly wrong," she said. "My baby is going to die."

Rachel ordered all the standard tests, with normal results. The only unusual signs were a slightly elevated respiration rate and half a degree of fever. Baffled, she asked her resident's permission to do a lumbar puncture, a painful test rarely performed unless there's clear evidence that meningitis might be the diagnosis. The resident scoffed. "Send them home," he said, and walked out.

But when Rachel tried to send the baby home, the mother burst into tears. "Please, doctor," she said, and Rachel suddenly just knew she was right. "One more test," she told the mother, and she did a lumbar puncture. She had just inserted a needle into the baby's spinal canal when the enraged resident burst in shouting, "What are you doing?" As she turned toward him, his expression changed. Looking back at the needle, she saw the first drop of pus flow through it. The baby had meningitis. If she had sent him home, he would have been dead within hours.

Rachel told me another story about unexplainable knowing from her personal life. When Rachel's father died, Rachel's elderly mother came to live with her. The house where Rachel was living was too small for the two of them and Rachel started looking for a bigger home. They had found a perfect house, a duplex, shared by a lovely older woman. It was spacious with beautiful views and seemed just right to Rachel.

But Rachel's mother didn't think so. Once a powerful, professional woman in her own right, at 80 she had become absent-minded and forgetful and sometimes confused. Still she was usually supportive of Rachel's decisions as she had been all of Rachel's life. But even before entering the house she had said, "We cannot live here."

Rachel was surprised. "Why not, Mom?" she asked. "It is perfect for us." But her mother kept saying over and over, "We cannot live here," without offering a reason for her strong objection. This made no sense to Rachel and she continued to bring up all the pluses of this new home. Finally her mother took Rachel's arm. In an urgent voice she said, "We cannot LIVE here, Rachel. We cannot *LIVE* in this house." So Rachel gave up and eventually they found another home.

A few months later, a violent storm hit the area, causing extensive flooding, many mudslides, and much structural damage. The duplex Rachel loved so was in the path of a huge mudslide and destroyed. Fortunately, the older woman occupying the other side of the house was not home at the time, but Rachel and her mother were at home . . . and safe in their new house. They would have certainly been injured if not killed had they rented the duplex.

Another physician friend told me his own experience of feeling guided at work in a way that felt purposeful and protective. Sean was a medical resident, still learning the skills doctors need in order to feel confident in emergency situations, when he found himself struggling to access the radial artery of a patient in shock in order to insert a line into it. The patient's arteries were clamped down from shock, and Sean could not thread the guide wire that needed to go into the narrow blood vessel. After many futile attempts, Sean became panicked, looking around for help and finding no one, knowing that this critical step was necessary to save the patient's life.

Then something came over Sean, and he found himself stepping back from the patient's bed and closing his eyes. A sense of peace overtook him, and he did something he had never done. He asked the Universe for help. He didn't really know who he was asking, but he heard a voice say, "Go ahead."

He thanked the voice and felt energized and reassured. When he opened his eyes and stepped up to the patient, without doubt, hesitation, or difficulty, Sean was able to access the patient's radial artery immediately, and the patient's life was saved.

Thinking back on it, Sean said, "It felt as though my hand was guided into the right place by an external force, and this phenomenon gave me a sense of amazement and awe. This was the first time I really felt connected to another level, a benevolent force. Since then, I've felt this guidance many, many times when helping to provide solutions to my patients. I firmly believe we have access to a whole other level in order to help each other, and I believe that our universe is indeed a friendly place that we create on an ongoing basis."

I was talking to my friend Tosha Silver about how guidance like this shows up, and she referred me to a story in her book *Outrageous Openness.* In one of the many stories she shares about letting the Divine take the lead, she writes about her straitlaced, highly skeptical economics professor friend Don, who liked to introduce Tosha as his "wacky psychic pal with a degree from Yale." One day, Tosha asked him, "Really, Don, total truth. Has anything ever happened that made you wonder if you had the full picture? Anything ever rock your perfect little rational world?"

Don went on to tell her about one night when he was in college, when he went to sleep before his roommate had come home for the night. At 3 A.M., Don awoke with a pounding heart and heard his roommate calling his name—twice. But the room was empty. He put on his clothes, stumbled out to his VW Bug, and started driving, only it was more like the car was driving itself. Don was drawn, like a magnet, to a spot ten blocks away, where he found his roommate buried under a snowbank, drunk, disoriented, and freezing.

Tosha was fascinated. "Man, you gotta be kidding me. This didn't change your life at all?"

Don said, "No way. I had to see it all as a coincidence. If I hadn't, I would have had to question everything."

When such things happen, people tend to either respond the way Lisby did and conclude "This changes everything" or sweep it under the carpet the way Don did. But I'm a little baffled about why people would deny such experiences. Perhaps they're afraid of what they don't understand. Personally, I find that stories like this actually make me less afraid, because they affirm my worldview: in a purposeful universe, we don't need to always be on guard against a dangerous world.

I wondered if other people had experiences of intuitive knowing that left them feeling comforted and less afraid. I sought out stories from my friends and colleagues, my online community, my blog readers, Facebook, and Twitter. I asked people to tell me about anything they had personally experienced that made them believe they lived in a purposeful universe. Over five hundred people submitted their stories of how they knew things they couldn't have known, and because of what they intuitively knew, saved someone's life—or their own. They told stories of telepathic messages they received from loved ones in danger, intuitive knowing that alerted them to trouble, and messages in dreams that solved problems and offered protection. They talked about what they considered miracles—people who appeared at just the right time, unexplainable cures for seemingly incurable illnesses, miraculous guidance that saved lives, and visitations from beings beyond this world.

I can't prove that the stories those in my online community shared with me are real, but they had the ring of truth to them. You could sense from those who told their stories how profoundly they were moved by their experiences and how much these experiences grew their faith. I could relate to how these people seemed to feel because I have seen the evidence too.

MY EVIDENCE FOR A PURPOSEFUL UNIVERSE

I was about eight years old, vacationing in North Carolina with my parents, where we were camping on the plot of land owned by my grandparents. It was autumn, and the fall leaves were raining their yellows and oranges across the landscape, but unusual weather resulted in fewer than usual of the bright crimson maple leaves my mother cherished. Planning to wax the fall leaves and decorate our table, Mom sent us out into the woods in search of the rare bright-red leaves, but I couldn't find a single one. I walked for what felt like miles along the yellow and brown leaf-lined dirt paths, until finally, I spotted a red one, high on a branch that hung over a steep cliff.

Longing to impress my mother with my spectacular find, I shimmied out on the tree limb, perched over the steep cliff, and plucked the bright-red leaf off the branch, just as the branch cracked. I spilled down the hillside, dropping my red leaf. I was spared from plummeting onto the rocks below by a small shrub I was able to grab.

There I was using all of my eight-year-old strength to cling to that shrub, when a man with a warm, loving smile on his face appeared above me. Without saying a word, he gazed down at me, then lowered his walking stick over the edge. I don't know how I managed to grab onto that stick without falling, but I did, and the man pulled me up the hill. When I turned to thank him, he had vanished. I ran up and down the road, calling for him, but he never appeared again.

When I told Mom my story, she told me I had just been blessed with a miracle, that God had sent an angel to save my life. I was less concerned about angels than about disappointing my mother by failing to bring home the beautiful red leaf that had fluttered away when the tree branch broke.

Then Mom said, "What's that?" She pulled something out of my pocket.

It was the red leaf.

Was this experience "real" or not? Perhaps rather than being saved by an angel, I was rescued by a hiker who just walked faster than me and managed to slip away before I noticed him. Maybe I hallucinated the whole thing. Jeffrey Kripal, Ph.D., a religious studies professor at Rice University who studies mystical experiences, suggests that perhaps we need not ask whether such experiences are "real" or "unreal." He proposes that we consider a third category—one that leaves room for the metaphoric and symbolic. He suggests that if a mystical experience offers guidance, eases fear, provides comfort, or expands consciousness, that is enough. Either way, the experience left my eight-year-old self with a conviction that there are things in this world—unseen things—that guide and protect us, and because of this, I don't need to live in fear.

As I grew older, I had other experiences that affirmed my worldview. Like many of the physicians Lisby interviewed, I started knowing things I shouldn't have known, things that seemed to protect my patients. One day, in the emergency room when I was a medical resident, a pregnant patient came in with what looked like the flu. All of her blood tests were normal, and I had no reason to believe anything else was wrong with her. My attending physician wanted to send her home, but for reasons I couldn't explain, I just knew her baby was in danger. I recommended a test that my teacher thought was crazy—an amniocentesis to assess the amniotic fluid around the baby. For some reason, my attending trusted my intuition and let me do the test. It turned out the amniotic fluid was infected with a bacteria that would have killed the baby had we not diagnosed it early enough to deliver the baby prematurely and start her on antibiotics.

I began getting other information that didn't come from my cognitive mind. I would be talking to someone I'd just met when I would sense something about the person that I couldn't have known and didn't have a way to verify as true. I'd sense that someone had been sexually molested as a child. Or I'd get a feeling that she was worried she would be laid off from her job or that she was thinking about leaving her husband. Later, the person would confide in me and confirm what I had sensed. It wasn't something I could rely on; sometimes I would get this kind of information, and often I would not. But the information I did get often seemed to be helpful in easing the suffering of my patients.

One day, when I was hiking, I saw a waking vision, like a movie being played on an invisible movie screen in front of me: I was sitting on the floor of my guest house, my back against a wall, with my client April lying in my arms, the back of her head resting on my chest. The movie was very specific—a lit candle, a crystal in April's hand, the scent of a specific aromatherapy oil. A voice-over said, "If you do this, she'll get better."

To my rational mind, the vision I saw was just plain crazy. First of all, April was my client. What I saw would be completely inappropriate for the kind of relationship we had. Second, as you know from reading her story earlier, April was a bodyguard with post-traumatic stress disorder who couldn't turn her back to anyone. Asking her to lie with her back to me would be insane. Third, I was not exactly the crystal-using kind of doctor. I didn't even *own* a crystal.

I wasn't sure what I was seeing. Was I making this all up? Was it just my imagination? Or was it something else? What if the voice-over I heard was true? What if I recreated what I saw in the vision and April's health problems got better? April was dealing with a variety of different chronic health conditions, most notably a rare type of anemia no hematologist had ever been able to properly diagnose, and she spent days every month connected to intravenous lines for infusions her doctors said she would require for the rest of her life.

As crazy as it sounded, I had experienced enough strange intuitive experiences with positive outcomes that I was coming to trust my intuition. I decided to run it by April. She agreed to try it, so we set up a session. The results shocked both of us, as well as her physician. It has now been over three years since April last got an infusion, and her blood count has been normal ever since.

I can't explain how I knew what I knew, and I certainly can't explain why April's anemia was cured. As Sir Arthur Eddington said, "Something unknown is doing we don't know what." Whatever it was, the experience changed us both.

After this experience—and after reading Lisby's book—I found myself becoming increasingly curious about the science of anomalous cognition. As a cognitive doctor, I had little inclination to meander into that fuzzy realm, much less to include a discussion of it in my book. But I was intrigued by the idea that intuition might be the vehicle through which the spirit realm communicates with the human realm. When life is confusing and we're having a hard time making decisions, perhaps we humans get guided toward the highest good by spiritual forces via our intuition. Wouldn't it be comforting if this were true? Might knowing that you're always being guided by well-meaning spiritual influences make you less afraid?

I started interviewing more people about their personal experiences of extraordinary knowing, and what struck me was that those who had come to trust their intuition were capable of taking great risks because they could sense whether or not the risk taking was aligned with their highest good. It can be a fine line between fearless and reckless, but these people didn't strike me as reckless. The people I interviewed who had cultivated and learned to trust their intuition felt like they were always being guided, and they were supported by this guidance more than they were controlled by their fears. One woman's story in particular struck me as an example of how difficult decisions can be made when you trust your intuition and the guidance of a purposeful universe.

A CURE BEYOND FEAR

When Kathleen was diagnosed with cervical cancer, her doctor wanted to schedule her for surgery right away. Kathleen wasn't at all surprised about the cancer. Intuitively, she had known something was wrong, so the diagnosis only confirmed what she had already sensed. Six months earlier, she, along with her husband and three sons, had left the spiritual commune that had been their home for 12 years. The story of why they left was the stuff of bad made-for-TV movies. But once they escaped and moved to Los Angeles, things began to unravel. Kathleen lost all patience with her kids and worried that she had become a bad mother. She had trouble controlling her anger and was afraid she might hurt her children. She knew she had to get away to work on healing herself. Even though she was terrified about abandoning her family, she finally told her husband she needed to leave for a while—to decompress so she could come back and be a good mother and wife. Her husband begged her not to go, but Kathleen's intuition insisted. Leaving her family behind, she moved to Mt. Shasta, which was reputed to be full of healing energies believed to rejuvenate the body and soul. She thought Mt. Shasta might be able to help her reclaim herself.

That's when her doctor called her to tell her she had cancer. According to the doctor, the pathology slides had been reviewed by two labs. The diagnosis was unequivocal. The doctor insisted she come back to Los Angeles and get surgery right away. But Kathleen *just knew* she wasn't supposed to get the surgery. She felt a keen intuition that she would die if she did. The idea that she might refuse cancer treatment sounded crazy to Kathleen's cognitive mind. Her doctor had warned her about what could happen if she refused to act right away with aggressive treatment. The cancer could spread and other organs could be affected. The doctor assured her that there was no way the cancer could go away on its own. Refusing treatment was a death sentence.

Kathleen was frightened. She really didn't want to die. But the voice of her intuition was stronger than the voice of her fear, so she decided against the surgery, because deep down, she just knew that the cancer was only the symptom. Her inner wisdom told her that if she didn't heal the underlying causes of her illness, the cancer would just come back.

Her doctor had explained that her cancer was most likely related to infection with the human papillomavirus, a virus known to transform healthy cervical cells into cancer. But Kathleen suspected it was more than that. The cancer was just a manifestation of something deeper. Perhaps the virus had caused her cancer, but she sensed that she had been susceptible to the virus because of an unhealed emotional wound that weakened her immune system and predisposed her to it. Her intuition told her that she had to heal the emotional wound first. After that, if the cancer was still there, she would get the surgery. She worried about how much she was upsetting her husband, but she was even more afraid that if she didn't do this, her family would lose her anyway. She dove into her healing journey with both feet.

Kathleen set about creating a treatment plan aimed at healing her mind's illness, while also tending to the needs of her body with holistic treatments. Putting her health into the hands of her intuitive knowing, Kathleen carefully sought out a team of practitioners to support her. Holistic health care providers recommended herbal tinctures, supplements, diet changes, and tai chi. Kathleen felt deeply nurtured by them, but she suspected what they were offering wasn't enough to cure her. They focused mostly on external treatments, and Kathleen's intuition kept coming back to the emotional wound she knew she'd have to face.

Then she met Joseph, who does deep-tissue bodywork meant to release not only the physiological knots in the muscles, but also the emotional blocks held in those knots. When Joseph began massaging Kathleen, she felt the breaking of a reservoir of fear-laced rage. Writhing on the massage table, nauseated and sobbing,

Kathleen moved through her anger and fear. The knotted mass of who she had become began to slowly and deeply unwind.

Between sessions, Kathleen went to the gym, took walks up the mountain, and cried in her room over how much she missed her three sons. Then one day, in the sauna at the gym, she met Kandis, a therapist who used a technique for healing the immune system aimed at identifying the moment in time when a life-negating decision is made. The goal of the treatment is to first release pent-up emotions of anger, guilt, and fear, then create a new life-affirming choice meant to activate the immune system.

Kathleen's work with Kandis began as talk therapy, aimed at ferreting out the major wounding events in Kathleen's life. Next, Kandis used kinesiology testing to see which of these events was directly weakening Kathleen's immune system, allowing her cancer to take hold. The muscle testing only further confirmed what Kathleen had already intuitively sensed about her past.

Kathleen had been only 15 when she found out she was pregnant. Nine months later, she was 16, lying in a hospital bed alone, wracked with labor pains. Suddenly, there was an emergency. Without asking her permission, the hospital staff grabbed her legs and tied them to the stirrups. Kathleen panicked, feeling violated. The doctor announced that he needed to do an episiotomy. Before she could consent, two nurses held her down by the shoulders. As she bucked, trying to get away, she felt large hands thrusting inside of her, then the agony of cutting through flesh.

It worked. The baby boy she was planning to give up for adoption slid out.

While sharing this story with Kandis, Kathleen suddenly understood why it wasn't just any cancer her weakened immune system allowed to manifest. It was her cervix, the portal through which that abandoned baby had come. It all made perfect sense. She hated her reproductive organs. She hated herself for giving up her baby. She knew she would have to heal this too.

Kandis took Kathleen to a mirror and invited her to look into the eyes of her teenage self. She instructed her to offer compassion to that young girl for what she had been through. Kathleen could feel the emotions of the loss all over again—the confusion, the tensions in her family, the agony of the birth, the love for the baby, the despair of the loss. The emotions felt almost too overwhelming to bear, but somehow, she was able to open her heart to that hurting teenager. After that session, Kathleen knew she had been healed.

By this point, it had been six months since she had moved to Mt. Shasta. Kathleen knew it was time to go home. She returned to Los Angeles and asked her doctor to biopsy her cervix.

The cancer was gone, and it never came back.

I was fascinated by Kathleen's story. The cognitive physician part of me thought her decision to refuse conventional cancer treatment was pretty reckless. Why would someone risk her life when she was a mother with young children who had a potentially curable cancer that responds well to treatment? Yet somehow, Kathleen just knew everything would be okay if she took an unconventional course.

Few people I meet in everyday life trust their intuition enough to let it make tough decisions the way Kathleen did. Instead, they're motivated by fear, and they let fear make their decisions because they think fear protects them. Kathleen trusted something else more than she trusted fear, and it resulted in a spontaneous remission from cancer. I started to wonder what would happen if more of us learned how to tune in to our intuition and trust the guidance we get from this inner compass. Would it be safe to make decisions in this way? Is intuition something we all have? Is there any evidence that all of us might have ways of knowing things we shouldn't know? My scientist brain wanted to know, and I had a feeling my answers might lie in the data reviewed in Lisby's book.

As I pondered the link between intuition and fear, I grew more convinced that anomalous cognition and courage were somehow related. If fear arises because of the limiting belief that we live in a dangerous world, and if courage stems from the trust that we're always being guided and protected in a purposeful universe, anomalous cognition may offer a bridge that allows Universal Intelligence to guide us meaningfully via our own intuition. Perhaps "psychic" abilities aren't just the province of people in muumuus with crystal balls. Maybe all of us can cultivate and learn to trust this kind of intuitive knowing that can help us make safe, healthy, courageous decisions. Is there evidence that my theory is true? As a scientist, I don't tend to take things like this on blind faith. I like evidence, and in case you do too, I'll share some of the scientific data suggesting that extraordinary knowing may be something real and available to us all.

SCIENTIFIC EVIDENCE OF ANOMALOUS COGNITION

In the 1930s, J. B. Rhine, Ph.D., and his wife, Louisa Rhine, Ph.D., pioneered the study of anomalous cognition at Duke University. The Rhines established the Rhine Research Center, and it is still run today by their daughter, Sally Rhine Feather, Ph.D. In 1948, Louisa Rhine began collecting letters written by people who were describing their experiences of extraordinary knowing. Her criteria for including these letters in her database required that the storyteller appear to be sharing the story in good faith, be of sound mind, and supply concrete factual information not available through any of the conventional five senses. She favored stories with extensive detail. Although she received over 30,000 letters, fewer than half of these made the cut for her database.

While Louisa Rhine was more interested in the stories, which provided a glimpse into a realm of experiences that she deemed difficult to explain away as mistakes of testimony, overinterpretation, imagination, coincidence, or lunacy, her husband was more interested in the science of precognition, which is defined as the ability to foresee an event before it happens, to essentially glimpse the future. J. B. Rhine's research focused on studying ordinary individuals who claimed no unusual abilities, using conventional scientific methods and procedures. Their primary goal was to definitively determine, using rigorously controlled scientific methodology, whether or not anomalous mental capacities could be proven to exist.

Researchers used a deck of 25 specially designed cards created by Karl Zener. Each card portrayed one of five simple geometric designs—a star, a square, wavy lines, a circle, and a plus sign. Two types of tests were performed. One tested clairvoyance, asking subjects to name a card that no other knew had been flipped up. The second type of experiment tested telepathy, and subjects were asked to name a card another person was thinking of. A correct guess was deemed a "hit." With 25 cards, pure chance would predict that people would guess 5 correctly. The researchers wanted to see if their subjects could outperform chance. After three years and 100,000 tests with ordinary research participants, the Rhines were able to demonstrate positive and statistically significant results well beyond chance, which suggested that anomalous mental capacities were indeed possible within the ordinary population.[4]

Their research led them to a young divinity student, Hubert E. Pearce, Jr., who far outperformed ordinary individuals in his ability to predict the cards. Pearce was studied by Rhine's research assistant Joseph Pratt. Pratt and Pearce would separate themselves by distance—Pratt in the Duke physics building and Pearce in the Duke library—and after they synchronized their watches, Pratt would shuffle a deck of these "Zener cards," pick the top card off the deck, and lay it facedown on the table in front of him. Meanwhile, Pearce would write down which card he thought Pratt was laying down. A minute later, Pratt would pick another card and repeat this procedure until all 25 cards were turned over. Then he'd shuffle the cards and start over again. The two men conducted 1,850 trials, during which Pearce correctly guessed the right cards 558 times. Pure chance would have him guessing correctly 370 times. The odds that Pearce would correctly guess 558 cards out of 1,850 were 22 billion to 1.

Based on the Pearce-Pratt experiments, Rhine coined a new term—*extra-sensory perception,* or ESP. In 1934, Rhine published *Extra-Sensory Perception,* which was widely embraced by the public and reached millions of readers. As the first real scientist rigorously testing anomalous cognition, Rhine's data made quite a splash in both the academic world and in the press. News media and popular journals like *The New York Times* and *Scientific American* snatched it up. Academic institutions called the research "epoch-making." And anomalous cognition made its way into university psychology classes.

But then controversy erupted. A series of assaults plagued Rhine and his research. Critics claimed that his data was methodologically flawed. The Rhines took the critiques of their methods to heart and redesigned their studies. Much of the critique revolved around "sensory leakage"—ways in which the ordinary five senses might have "leaked" to subjects and influenced the cards they chose. In response, the Rhines replaced the human card shufflers with machines and isolated all subjects in separate locations from the testers, making them incapable of getting clues from sensory leakage. In 1937, the American Institute of Mathematics proclaimed the lab's procedures and statistical methods fully valid.

In 1938, the Rhine research was critiqued in a public debate forum at the convention of the American Psychological Association. Rhine, as well as Gardner Murphy and one of Rhine's statisticians, met with resounding applause after fielding the debate questions. By all accounts, Rhine had the support of his colleagues.

But controversy once again plagued Rhine when he published his follow-up book, *Extra-Sensory Perception After Sixty Years,* or *ESP-60* as it came to be known. Initially the book appeared on Harvard's required reading lists for the introductory psychology classes. But soon thereafter, Rhine's book was denounced as "pseudoscience" and disappeared from college reading lists. After that, the American Psychological Association stopped talking publicly about ESP and other anomalous mental capacities. In spite of the public's widespread curiosity about his work, Rhine's lab settled into scientific obscurity, with its data published only in the obscure *Journal of Parapsychology.* In her book *The Gift,* Sally Feather Rhine discusses the current status of the Rhine lab and says, "Our efforts today no longer focus on whether ESP exists; we have strong evidence that it does." Yet, here we are, living in a world of scientists and rationalists who raise eyebrows if you suggest that precognition is real.

The mainstream world of science still dismisses the existence of anomalous cognition. But if you look at the scientific data objectively, and if you honor the experiences of everyday people, it's hard not to conclude that anomalous cognition is real. Can I prove it without a doubt? No. Why is this? If anomalous cognition is a real human ability, why isn't the scientific data more conclusive? I have to wonder whether our scientific methods of determining what is "real" are simply too limited to verify all the mysteries of the universe. Maybe intuition isn't meant to be used to predict cards. Maybe that's not purposeful enough. Maybe it's reserved for what really matters—anticipating danger, protecting those we love, intuiting when it's time to leave a relationship, or knowing how to make the right medical treatment decisions. All I can say is that my intuition has saved me many times, and it has helped me protect others, and somehow, this makes me feel safer and more capable of taking risks.

TRAGEDY IN A PURPOSEFUL WORLD

I wouldn't be a real scientist if I didn't acknowledge what some might view as evidence that flies in the face of the idea of a purposeful universe. How can we say it's not a dangerous world when our world has been through the Holocaust or the Rwanda genocide? What about incest and school shootings and child abductions and children who get cancer? What about women sold into sexual slavery and natural disasters that devastate communities? What about wars that kill innocent people? How can a purposeful universe allow such atrocities?

The honest answer is I don't know. That's the thing about life's purpose. It's all a mystery. Suggesting that it's a purposeful universe doesn't mean that things will always work out the way we want. As spirits having a human experience, we have free will, and because we're human, we're prone to mistakes. Inner and outer guidance is always available to us, but too often, we ignore it. We violate it. We sell our souls in order to get what our Small Selves desire. When this happens, suffering ensues. I can only imagine that our creator weeps as we destroy our environment and inflict genocide upon one another. Surely, our creator hopes we wake up soon.

It's so tempting to think we know what's "good" or "bad" and to get upset when things don't go our way. But perhaps our purposeful universe isn't so black-and-white. For example, California has been in the midst of a terrible drought, ostensibly as a result of human-inflicted climate change. The fires have been burning through the state, and the animals are dying. A friend of mine suggested that we need to gather in ceremony to do a rain dance and pray for relief from the drought. It's easy to assume that the "best" thing would be a giant rainstorm. But what if that's not what's best? What if our purposeful universe has a grander plan, and it's actually more aligned for California to get so dry that wildfires burn homes to the ground in order to wake us up to the gravity of how much we're destroying our planet? Maybe devastation from drought will help us turn things around before it's too late to save ourselves. Or maybe not.

Considering such things raises more questions than answers. Why is one person gifted with a premonition that saves a child's life, while another has no such knowing and gets blindsided by a child's seemingly senseless death? Why does one person experience a miraculous healing from a terminal disease, while another dies? If there is a Universal Intelligence that guides and protects us, why doesn't it intervene to prevent genocide, war, and violence against children?

Philosophers and theologians have pondered such questions for millennia and there are many beliefs, but none can be proven. We have to keep trusting that if we live in a purposeful universe in which we are unconditionally loved, there must be a reason for even the most seemingly senseless losses we experience. We are not at the mercy of a random, chaotic universe. We are not being punished because of our imperfections or spiritual disobedience. We are not being thrown to the proverbial wolves because we're not worthy of grace. This means we must trust that whatever happens, it is purposeful, and we will someday be granted insight into the nature of what happens in life.

As Steve Jobs said in his famous commencement speech at Stanford in 2005, "You can't connect the dots looking forward. You can only connect them looking backwards. So you have to trust that the dots will somehow connect in your future. You have to trust in something: your gut, destiny, life, karma, whatever. Because believing that the dots will connect down the road will give you the confidence to follow your heart, even when it leads you off the well-worn path."

Once you realize that nothing is random, that you weren't the victim of bad luck or bad genes or hostile forces, that even illnesses and those who hurt you were teachers of your soul and deserving of gratitude, you're ready to transform your relationship with fear and uncertainty. Once you make the essential choice to trust that the universe is a purposeful place, you may find that you are less afraid of all that you have to lose, because you're willing to lose everything if it's aligned with this greater purpose. You no longer think it's your job to protect and guard and armor up, because you know that life unarmored is filled with so much more love and intimacy. Trusting that you live in a purposeful universe opens the portal so you can come into right relationship with uncertainty. You can lean into uncertainty, open to mystery with wonder and awe, rather than avoiding risk or uncertainty at all costs. You open yourself to the unearned blessings of grace, and something shifts. This changes everything. You are gifted with courage and can take right action, claiming your place in this purposeful universe.

Walter Kohn, the American theoretical physicist who was awarded the Nobel Prize in 1998, said, "I have been influenced in my thinking by the writing of Einstein who has made remarks to the effect that when he contemplated the world he sensed an underlying Force much greater than any human force. I feel very much the same. There is a sense of awe, a sense of reverence, and a sense of great mystery."

Perhaps we're meant to lean into the mystery without understanding it all. Perhaps this is where we truly become brave.

COURAGE-CULTIVATING EXERCISE #9

Consider the Evidence

1. Take a moment and consider whether you've ever
    experienced something extraordinary or unexplain-
    able, something that doesn't quite make sense to the
    cognitive mind. Have you had your own harp story?
    Have you ever known something you shouldn't have
    known? Have you predicted some future outcome in a
    dream? Has someone called you right when you were
    thinking about him or her? Have you been seized by
    an unexplainable impulse to do something that wound
    up helping another person who was in crisis? Have
    you *just known* where to find a lost object? Have you
    diagnosed someone's illness or foreseen someone's
    death before it happened? Have you communicated
    telepathically with a person or animal? Have you
    acted on a premonition that wound up protecting you
    or someone else? Have you seen visions, heard voices,
    or experienced guidance you can't otherwise explain?
    Have you experienced synchronicities you can't write
    off as mere coincidence? Reflect upon your past and
    consider whether you've ever felt guided, either by
    your own intuition, another person's guidance, or
    external "signs from the Universe," in a way that pro-
    tected you or someone else from harm.

2. Make a list of all of these experiences—your own per-
    sonal evidence that you live in a purposeful universe.

3. For each experience you've written down, con-
    sider how you responded to this experience. Did
    you ignore it? Did you rationalize it away? Did you
    trivialize it and write it off as coincidence? Do you
    make up implausible stories to explain it? Did you
    tell others your story? Did you keep your experience
    a secret? Did you have a "This changes everything"
    moment? Or did nothing change?

For assistance with this process, visit TheFearCureBook.com and
download the free Prescription for Courage Kit, which includes
a guided meditation meant to guide you in a reflection that will
help you recall evidence that you live in a purposeful universe.

COURAGE-CULTIVATING EXERCISE #10

Find Meaning in Everything

We may never fully understand why things happen the way they do, but when we shift how we perceive what happens, especially when we're in the midst of something that feels scary, we realize that it's possible to find meaning in even the most seemingly meaningless events. You can apply this practice whenever you find yourself spiraling into victimhood.

1. Imagine that your soul and Universal Intelligence sat down before you were born and made a plan to craft your life in such a way that you learn certain lessons in this lifetime. For example, if your soul came here to learn self-reliance, you might pick a family that would leave you an orphan. If you came here to learn to handle rejection with grace, you might wind up dumped by multiple lovers. If you came here to make peace with uncertainty, you might wind up with a life-threatening illness.

2. Based on your current life challenge, what might your soul be learning? Why might your soul and Universal Intelligence have agreed to co-create this situation? What lessons are you learning?

3. Bless the situation. Express gratitude to those who might be teaching you these lessons. Thank the challenge for all you're learning.

COURAGE-CULTIVATING EXERCISE #11

Ask to Be Shown

Not sure you believe it's a purposeful universe? Not feeling guided? Never experienced something that leaves you wondering if there might be more? Feeling doubtful about whether a divine presence even exists? Sometimes those of us with very cognitive minds need evidence. Try a little experiment. Whatever it is you trust—whether it's God, Buddha, Mohammed, Pachamama, or your Inner Pilot Light—try asking for evidence of a purposeful universe or guidance in a way you'll be able to clearly identify. Be as specific or general as feels right for you. Then be sure to release attachment to any outcome. If you get obsessed about grasping for evidence or guidance, the clutching energy can interfere with the flow of guidance, so it's important not to make the quest for guidance yet another goal the Small Self can obsess about.

After you do this, pay close attention to your dreams, be on the lookout for synchronicities, notice messages that appear in books, on billboards, or on license plates, listen to your intuition, call upon all your senses to spot the guidance that's always trying to reach us, and stay alert for evidence of a purposeful universe. Keep in mind that this is not about making demands on the Divine. It's an offering, an invitation to the Divine to help you grow your trust. If you don't get a sign, don't despair. You haven't been abandoned. Your guidance will come. Be patient and trust that your guidance will arrive in divine timing in the perfect way.

CHAPTER 7

WE ARE ALL ONE

You and I are all as much continuous with the physical universe as a wave is continuous with the ocean.

— ALAN WILSON WATTS

After walking on the moon, the sixth man ever to do so, Apollo 14 astronaut Edgar Mitchell approached Earth from outer space, and as he gazed at the beautiful blue planet we call home, he was struck with an experience of the Oneness of all things—a profound, euphoric sense of interconnectedness with all of life. He felt a certainty that he was returning to part of a living system, harmonious and whole—and that we all participate, as he later expressed it, "in a universe of consciousness." Mitchell has said that this experience transformed him from one fascinated by exploring outer space to one committed to understanding "inner space." Although he was trained as an engineer, scientist, and astronaut, Mitchell journeyed back from outer space with a sense of inner knowing that radically altered his worldview. Despite science's great advances, he realized that we had barely touched the universe's greatest mystery.

Mitchell said, "What I do remember is the awesome experience of recognizing the universe was not simply random happenstance . . . that there was something more operating than just chance." Seeing Earth from space, he no longer felt the sense of separation he had felt his whole life, that sense of "I" and "they." Instead, he returned from space with an understanding that all the humans, animals, and systems on the planet were a part of one synergistic whole.

Within two years of his journey into outer space, Edgar Mitchell founded the Institute of Noetic Sciences (IONS) in 1973. The IONS vision statement reads, "We encourage open-minded explorations of consciousness through the meeting of science and spirit. We take inspiration from the great discoveries of human history that have been sourced from insight and intuition and that have harnessed reason and logic for their outer expression. It is our conviction that systematic inquiries into consciousness will catalyze positive concrete transformations in the world. In this process, our vision is to help birth a new worldview that recognizes our basic interconnectedness and interdependence and promotes the flourishing of life in all its magnificent forms."

The kind of shift in perspective that Mitchell experienced was termed the "overview effect" by Frank White, who investigated this phenomenon and transformed it into the book and documentary film both titled *The Overview Effect*. In the film, Mitchell talks about his "aha" moment when he looked out over the heavens and realized that every molecule in his body and every molecule in the bodies of the other astronauts in Apollo 14 were all made of stardust. He was confused by this spiritual epiphany, and after returning to Earth, he sought answers, first from books, and then from professors at a local university. He was told that the ancient literature described a state called *savikalpa samadhi,* which means, as he put it, that "you see things as you see them with your eyes, but you experience them emotionally and viscerally with ecstasy and a sense of total unity and Oneness."

Mitchell said, "Well, that's exactly what the experience was. And so it was clear to me as I studied this that it wasn't anything new, but it was something that was very important to the way we humans were put together."

AN INFINITE WHOLE

It's not just astronauts who have experienced epiphanies waking them up to this feeling of Oneness. Many people who have had near-death experiences report similar expansions of consciousness. Anita Moorjani, who experienced a spontaneous remission from stage 4 lymphoma after her near-death experience, told her story in *Dying to Be Me*. Her body was riddled with tumors, her organs were all shutting down, her lungs were filled with liquid, and Anita was unconscious when the doctors told her family she was dying.

But Anita was watching the whole thing from above as she simultaneously experienced the kind of rapturous feeling of Oneness the astronaut felt while looking back at Earth. Anita wrote, "I was overwhelmed by the realization that God isn't a being, but a state of being . . . and I was now that state of being!" With this new understanding, she explains, "I became aware that we're all connected. This was not only every person and living creature, but the interwoven unification felt as though it were expanding outward to include everything in the universe—every human, animal, plant, insect, mountain, sea, inanimate object, and the cosmos. I realized that the entire universe is alive and infused with consciousness, encompassing all of life and nature. Everything belongs to an infinite Whole. I was intricately, inseparably enmeshed with all of life."

Harvard neurosurgeon Eben Alexander, M.D., also experienced a sense of Oneness and unconditional love when he was in a coma, dying from E. coli meningitis. In his book *Proof of Heaven*, he reports a detailed journey into an altered state of consciousness, which he deemed "heaven." Based on his near-death experience, he came to the conclusion that we are all One. In the set of principles of consciousness and the cosmos that he distilled from his experience, called the Seven Cornerstone Postulates, he writes,

"All things in the cosmos are interconnected at the quantum level, influencing each other non-locally and instantaneously, implying that all things are one in the grand web of creation . . . In an interconnected universe, an infinite matrix of cause-effect relationships exists, suggesting that what we do to others we do to ourselves, which means that we reap what we sow . . . The good of the one and the good of the many are symbiotic, affirming the ancient wisdom that we can be only as strong as our weakest link."

A STROKE OF INSIGHT

Scientists are always trying to explain mystical experiences of Oneness such as these by coming up with rational explanations of what happens in the brain. They've posited that perhaps astronauts experience the overview effect because of some neurologic event that gets triggered at zero gravity. They've suggested that perhaps near-death experiences activate some part of the brain that simulates an experience of Oneness neurologically. Maybe they're right. Maybe the state of Oneness described by Eastern religions as *savikalpa samadhi* is nothing more than a trick of the brain. Neuroscientist Jill Bolte Taylor, Ph.D., had the opportunity to unwittingly perform an amazing personal experiment to assess whether such a theory could be true.

Having spent her career studying the brain, Dr. Taylor was well acquainted with the difference between the left and right hemispheres of the brain. In her famous TED talk, which at the time of this writing has been viewed more than 15 million times, Dr. Taylor explains that the right hemisphere is all about the present moment—right here, right now. The right hemisphere thinks in pictures, learns kinesthetically through the movement of the body, and streams in information through our senses before exploding into a collage of experiences that make up the present moment—what it looks like, smells like, tastes like, feels like, and sounds like.

Dr. Taylor says, "I am an energy being connected to the energy all around me through the consciousness of my right hemisphere.

We are energy beings connected to one another through the consciousness of our right hemispheres as one human family."

The left hemisphere, on the other hand, is a very different place. The left hemisphere thinks linearly and methodically and focuses on the past and the future. While it gets involved in the present moment, it does so only to break the vast collage of the present moment down into more and more details, categorizing all the input it receives. It analyzes the present moment by associating it with everything it has ever analyzed in the past, and it projects the present moment into the future by considering all of our possibilities of how things could play out.

The left hemisphere thinks in language, which shows up as the constant brain chatter of your Small Self, that analytical intelligence that's always barking out orders about what you did in the past and what you need to do in the future. Dr. Taylor says, "Perhaps most important, it's that little voice that says to me, 'I am. I am.' And as soon as my left hemisphere says to me 'I am,' I become separate. I become a single solid individual separate from the energy flow around me and separate from you."

This left hemisphere, the part that feeds into the fourth Fearful Assumption, "I am all alone," is the part of the brain that Dr. Taylor lost on the morning of her stroke. As the stroke was happening, Dr. Taylor noticed how different she felt inside. "At first I was shocked to find myself inside of a silent mind. But then I was immediately captivated by the magnificence of energy around me. And because I could no longer identify the boundaries of my body, I felt enormous and expansive. I felt at one with all the energy that was, and it was beautiful there."

Flickers of her left brain came back online and alerted her to the need to get help. She knew something wasn't quite right. Then her left brain flickered off and she drifted into that expansive space again. "Imagine what it would be like to be totally disconnected from your brain chatter that connects you to the external world," she says. "Any stress related to my job, it was gone. And I felt lighter in my body. And imagine all of the relationships in the external world and the many stressors related to any of those. They were gone . . . And imagine what it would feel like to lose

37 years of emotional baggage! . . . I felt enormous and expansive, like a genie just liberated from her bottle. . . . I remember thinking there's no way I would ever be able to squeeze the enormousness of myself back inside this tiny little body.

"But I realized 'But I'm still alive! I'm still alive and I have found Nirvana. And if I have found Nirvana and I'm still alive, then everyone who is alive can find Nirvana.' I picture a world filled with beautiful, peaceful, compassionate, loving people who knew that they could come to this space at any time. And that they could purposely choose to step to the right of their left hemispheres and find this peace. And then I realized what a tremendous gift this experience could be, what a stroke of insight this could be to how we live our lives."

She concludes her TED talk by saying, "We have the power to choose, moment by moment, who and how we want to be in the world. Right here right now, I can step into the consciousness of my right hemisphere where we are—I am—the life force power of the universe, and the life force power of the fifty trillion beautiful molecular geniuses that make up my form. At one with all that is. Or I can choose to step into the consciousness of my left hemisphere, where I become a single individual, a solid, separate from the flow, separate from you . . . Which would you choose? Which do you choose? And when?"[1]

If your mind is full of thoughts like *I am all alone,* it's easy to be frightened. But after you've experienced the overview effect, a near-death experience, a left brain stroke, or any other experience of Oneness, you'll find yourself stripped of the *I am all alone* thought. In its place, "We are all One" emerges to comfort you and inspire you to take tender care of your fellow beings.

ONENESS AS AN ANTIDOTE FOR FEAR

How does Oneness apply to everyday life, and how does it relate to fear? To consider this question, think of being a child who is afraid of the dark. When we were children, most of us were frightened at some point when we were alone at night. Maybe your mother would ask you to go get something from your room at night, and in order to get there, you'd have to run through a dark hallway or up the stairs by yourself. You'd go bravely into the dark, turning on lights as you went, but at some point, you might get gripped by a panicky feeling that made you run faster. You'd imagine scary monsters that weren't real and you'd feel the world closing in on you. When you're a little child all by yourself, venturing into the darkness can be downright terrifying. But it's different if your best friend is there. You still have to face the dark unknown, but you can hold hands and venture into the darkness together. Somehow, just holding that one person's hand, knowing you don't have to face the darkness alone, makes it less scary.

Diving into life is like venturing into the dark. If you feel you're venturing into the vast unknown all by yourself, it can feel very scary to willingly put yourself out of your comfort zone. But if someone is there to hold your hand, whether they're with you in person or connected to you on some other plane, having the company of others who care about you tends to make you feel brave. When you hold the worldview that you're a separate, solitary human being, venturing into the darkness of life's uncertainties all by yourself, it's easy to feel lonely and scared. But when you sense that you are One with every other being on the planet and that you are somehow tuned in with those you love, especially if one of you is in danger, it makes a difference. I find this strangely comforting, and it makes me feel brave. It also makes me feel more compassion for my fellow human beings, even the ones I don't know. On some level, if we're all One, then any suffering being is also me suffering, and my heart must stay open to everyone in order to raise the vibration of us all.

In his book *One Mind,* Larry Dossey, M.D., describes Oneness as "a collective, unitary domain of intelligence, of which all individual minds are a part." He claims that awakening to One Mind awareness not only alleviates the illusion of separation that underlies all fear, but also "is a potential way out of the division, bitterness, selfishness, greed, and destruction that threaten to engulf our world—from which, beyond a certain point, there may be no escape. Identifying with the highest expressions of human consciousness can clear our vision, prevent the hardening of our moral and ethical arteries, and inspire us to action."

Is there such a thing as a collective consciousness, and if so, what is it? Might there be some sort of energy field of knowledge we can all tap into from time to time in order to exchange information without using the traditional five senses? If so, can we prove it? Certainly, stories of the experience of Oneness pop up over and over in the study of religion and philosophy, but does the idea of Oneness intersect with science? Are we really all connected? And if so, can this realization that we are all One comfort us and make us less frightened?

CONNECTION AND COMMUNICATION

In _A Brief History of Everything,_ Ken Wilber wrote, "Are the mystics and sages insane? . . . [They all tell the same] story of awakening one morning and discovering you are one with the All, in a timeless and eternal and infinite fashion." Meditating Buddhist monks, yogis, Catholic saints, the mystics of all religions, and people on shamanic journeys who take ayahuasca share similar stories as those who have traveled into space or almost died. But are such stories real? Yes, the stories keep showing up in personal anecdotes, but anecdotes don't make good science since, as Wilber suggests, we could dismiss them all as the fantasies of wishful thinkers or the delusions of lunatics. I was curious as to whether I could find any real scientific evidence validating the kind of Oneness described by those who report mystical experiences.

At first, I just found more stories. In _Extraordinary Knowing,_ Elizabeth Lloyd Mayer (aka "Lisby," if you recall) collected stories of her therapist colleagues who seemed to be telepathically communicating with clients. Susan Coates, Ph.D., the world authority on early childhood, told the story of treating a four-year-old girl whom she saw one October 2—a significant date because that was the anniversary of the death of Susan's brother, who had drowned at 25 while trying to save someone's life. Her young patient was playing, when suddenly, out of the blue, she turned to Susan and said, "Your brother is drowning—you have to save him!" The hair stood up on the back of Susan's neck. She said, "No one is going to drown because we will save them." Then the little girl went right back to playing. Susan said there was no logical way the child could have known that part of her story.

Paula Hamm, a psychoanalyst, shared her story of seeing an image in her mind of a toddler with a plastic bag over his head. She sensed a feeling of distress that accompanied the image. She didn't recognize the child or attach any meaning to the vision. She likely would have forgotten it if it weren't for the patient she saw two hours later, who started the session by telling the story of the distressing situation he'd just experienced. He had been preparing dinner when his little boy walked in with a plastic bag held tight around his neck. They got the bag off before it did any damage, but the man was shaken.

Robert Stoller, M.D., a professor of psychiatry at UCLA Medical School, had written a paper in 1973 called "Telepathic Dreams," but he was advised by his mentor, Ralph Greenson, never to publish it if he valued his reputation. Not long after he read Stoller's paper, Greenson shared with Stoller that his son Danny had lost control of a motorcycle in San Francisco and had been admitted to the hospital with a compound fracture of his left leg. Because of the injury, Danny, who was supposed to start medical school, might not be able to attend school on time.

Stoller was astonished. The same night Danny had been injured, Stoller had dreamed that he was back in San Francisco, where he'd done his internship, working in an emergency room on a medical student who had a compound fracture of his left leg. The dream was so vivid that he had told his own therapist about the dream, and his therapist had recorded its details before Stoller found out what happened to Greenson's son. This was the first of a series of bewildering events for Stoller that revolved around dreams. He started to notice a pattern. Patients started coming in after the weekend, reporting dreams that mirrored what Stoller had just experienced in his personal life, as if his patients were somehow unconsciously tuning in to what he had experienced.

For example, one of his patients described a dream about a party at someone's home. People were milling around a large room in which one whole wall was made of glass. Then an older man carrying a large object suddenly smashed through the glass. The old man wasn't hurt, but there was glass everywhere. Over the same weekend that the patient had this dream, Stoller had been at a party, where someone had given a speech. Afterward, Stoller had volunteered to help move chairs through the sliding glass doors on one side of the room, and, not recognizing that the glass door was closed, he had crashed right through it. The glass broke and scattered across the floor, but nobody was hurt.

In another dream, a different patient of Stoller's was walking through a house under construction. A sunken bath was being put into the bathroom, and someone had put an initial into the still-soft cement. Unbeknownst to the patient, Stoller was in the middle of building a house. That same weekend, Stoller discovered that someone had vandalized the newly installed sunken bath. In the drying cement, someone had inscribed an initial.

Such events kept happening with startling regularity, and Stoller collected notes for 13 years before his still-unpublished "Telepathic Dreams" paper wound up in Lisby's hands. The paper ended with these words: "Besides finding the whole subject of [telepathy] alien to my scientific beliefs, I have also hesitated to write this up because of not knowing if something right or wrong is going on in me. If, some day, it is found that such experiences reflect an ordinary enough function of human psychology, it will seem quaint that I was uneasy."

By the time Lisby read the copy of Stoller's paper, Stoller had died unexpectedly. Lisby reached out to his widow, who said that Stoller had finally overcome his uneasiness and was convinced that telepathy and other forms of unconscious communication were the most exciting frontier of Western science. He regretted having never pursued publication of his paper and had just gotten back to work on it when he died suddenly. Stoller's widow told Lisby she hoped to see her husband's paper finally published in a respectable scientific journal.

Lisby offered to help, and in 2001, the paper was published in the flagship journal of American psychoanalysis, the *Journal of the American Psychoanalytic Association,* along with Lisby's introduction and epilogue. The journal article evoked many comments and e-mails, mostly from people sharing their own experiences that they had kept secret until then. Lisby added their stories to her growing database.

After reading about experiences like Stoller's, I became curious whether anyone in my online community had had their own telepathic experiences. Many had. Clayton was in Rio de Janeiro for his brother Landon's wedding when, a few days after the ceremony, he and his family were all relaxing on the beach. Clayton's brother had walked down the beach alone about half an hour earlier when Clayton got a terrible, chilling feeling. He told his best friend, "Go find Landon! Go find Landon!" His friend took off down the beach. He finally got to Clayton's brother, where a lifeguard had just saved Landon from nearly drowning in the undertow.

Debra had attempted suicide, overdosing on medications, and was in intensive care when an old friend called her. They hadn't spoken for over a year. When she picked up the phone, he said simply, "Hey, how are you?" Assuming someone had alerted him to the suicide attempt, she asked who it was. He said nobody had called him—he had simply been overwhelmed with thoughts of her. He didn't know why he was calling. When she told him where she was, he started crying. He hadn't been able to explain why he couldn't get her off his mind. Now he knew.

Alexia had a similar experience. She called her mother, and when nobody picked up the phone, Alexia instantly knew her mother had taken pills and needed her help. Doubting herself, she tried calling two more times, but there was still no answer, so she jumped in a cab and found that her mother had taken a box of benzodiazepines. Alexia arrived in time to call an ambulance. Her mother pulled through and is still alive today.

With anecdote after anecdote about apparent telepathic communication, you have to wonder if we really are all connected in some way we can't fully measure or explain. The stories I was reading and hearing were compelling, and I found myself increasingly curious. But still, stories aren't science. My cognitive mind wanted more solid evidence. That's when I came across some real scientific data that suggests that perhaps we really are connected in ways we can't yet explain.

CLINICAL EVIDENCE OF ONENESS

People who report regularly experiencing anomalous cognition, such as those who self-identify as professional intuitives or psychics, often describe going in and out of a sort of trance state. They report calming down the cognitive mind and essentially tuning down the noise in order to tap into quieter realms of intuition and guidance. People who practice anomalous healing, such as "energy healing," describe the importance of getting into this same quiet state of receptivity. Yet, ordinary people participating in experiments with Zener cards in labs like the Rhine lab are not dropping into this trance state. Most of them are still firmly in their cognitive states of consciousness. Perhaps this limits how much science can measure anomalous cognition.

Researchers wondered whether there might be a way to simulate the receptivity people report experiencing in a trance state. Parapsychology researchers hypothesized that telepathic communication—defined as the ability to gather information about the thoughts, feelings, or activities of another person without the use of the ordinary five senses—might be more effective and more easily measured and validated if a sender was transmitting an image to a receiver who was asleep.

Although Freud was never willing to publicly announce his belief in telepathic communication, he did go as far as declaring it an "incontestable fact that sleep creates favorable conditions for telepathy."[2] Montague Ullman, M.D., a New York analyst at Maimonides Medical Center, agreed with Freud and, in 1961, Ullman decided to marry the new technology of the sleep laboratory with Freud's notion that the dream state improves the conditions for telepathy. A landmark study ensued, during which Ullman set out to determine whether someone acting as a "sender" could telepathically communicate with a sleeping "receiver," thereby influencing the content of the receiver's dream.

Receivers were hooked up to EEG machines that indicated when the receiver was in a REM cycle indicating the dream state. While the receiver slept, someone acting as the sender was alerted the minute the receiver entered REM sleep. The sender was then instructed to try to mentally transmit a visual image randomly selected from a large pool of images to the sleeping receiver. The receiver was awakened as soon as the REM cycle ended and asked to describe what he or she had been dreaming in as much detail as possible. Three independent judges were then asked to analyze the dream description, examine the original pool of images, and pick the image that most closely corresponded to the description of the sleeping receiver's dream. Over six years and 450 separate trials, the judges were able to choose the correct image that had been transmitted enough times that the overall odds of such a result were calculated to be less than 1 in 75 million.[3]

Such convincing numbers caused quite a stir in the world of sleep research. But unsurprisingly, there was no lack of skepticism. The study's methodology was rigorously examined by Irvin Child, Ph.D., at Yale, who verified that the study design was sound—but rational scientists have no mechanism to explain how such a thing could be possible, so resistance to even highly credited data was high.

Ullman was convinced that dream telepathy was real, that when people disengage from the cognitive mind during sleep, a natural capacity to transfer information from one person to another is freed up. This interested him on a societal level; he believed that this capacity reflected a powerful interconnectedness, showing how each individual's life was interwoven with others in the community, and that this may have offered a survival advantage from an evolutionary perspective.

Were his findings the scientific evidence I was seeking, validating the spiritual idea that we are all One? I was increasingly curious and wondered whether more scientific data might exist to support the notion of Oneness.

THE GANZFELD EXPERIMENTS

The dream telepathy work coming out of Ullman's Maimonides dream lab inspired the work of Charles Honorton, who had once struck up a correspondence with J. B. Rhine at Duke and later wound up working with Ullman at Maimonides, where he eventually became the director of the Division of Parapsychology and Psychophysics. In 1979, he founded the Psychophysical Research Laboratories at Princeton. Honorton had been interested in anomalous cognition since his teenage years, and his experience working in the sleep lab led him to wonder whether conditions could be created that would help turn down the mental noise of daily life in order to better study telepathy with *awake* people in a laboratory setting.

Researchers speculated that anomalous cognition might be available to all of us as a natural human capacity, but that perhaps its information showed up as weak signals that got drowned out by the noise of everyday life. They theorized that anomalous cognition might be better detected in a laboratory setting if study subjects were less distracted with everyday sensory stimuli. Honorton was curious whether it would be possible to minimize that mind noise so that any detectable telepathic influences might be amplified.

Along with parapsychology researchers William Braud, Ph.D., and Adrian Parker, Ph.D., Honorton went on to develop what came to be called the "ganzfeld" ("total field") method. The ganzfeld method involved inducing sensory deprivation in study subjects by taping translucent Ping-Pong ball halves over their eyes, directing a red floodlight toward the Ping-Pong balls, placing headphones over the subjects' ears, and playing white noise through the headphones. Subjects were then led through a series of relaxation exercises to help mute body sensations and mental chatter.

In the ganzfeld experiments, a "receiver" was outfitted with the Ping-Pong balls and earphones, while the "sender" was taken to a soundproof room at a distance and instructed to spend 30 minutes concentrating on a randomly selected image and focusing on transmitting it telepathically to the receiver. The receiver was instructed to spend those 30 minutes just thinking aloud, verbally describing any images or thoughts that came to mind in a stream-of-consciousness fashion. After the session was completed, the receiver was then shown four images, which included the one the sender was trying to transmit. The receiver was asked to rank the images based on how closely they corresponded to images or thoughts he or she had experienced during the 30-minute period. If the receiver chose the correct image, it counted as a "hit." If not, it was a "miss." The hit rate expected by chance was one in four, or 25 percent.

Honorton published a paper reviewing 42 separate ganzfeld telepathy experiments conducted by ten different experimenters from labs across the globe. The average hit rate was 35 percent. The odds of this outcome appearing from chance were calculated to be ten billion to one.[4]

The publication of this data caused quite a stir, arousing the attention of admitted skeptic Ray Hyman, a cognitive psychologist at the University of Oregon. Cynical about the data, Hyman decided to independently analyze the same data Honorton had analyzed.[5] In a scientifically collegial arrangement, Honorton and Hyman agreed that both would conduct separate meta-analyses on all previously published ganzfeld data and compare results. In 1986, they published their data in the *Journal of Parapsychology* and came to similar conclusions. While they differed as to whether their results provided solid proof that telepathy exists, they agreed that the data was real and couldn't be explained as either chance or methodological error.[6] Other researchers replicated these early ganzfeld studies, coming up with consistent hit rates in the 33–35 percent range, suggesting that telepathic communication between humans really is possible.

Critics were skeptical of the ganzfeld data, but it remained compelling, and scientists continued to pore over it. Lisby was one of them, intrigued by the findings. As she wrote, "This, finally, was starting to look like science." One article published in the major peer-reviewed journal *Psychological Bulletin* concluded that the ganzfeld data provides solid, replicable data that telepathy exists.[7] Another article, also published in *Psychological Bulletin*, concludes just as resoundingly that telepathy doesn't exist.[8]

The question of whether or not we can trust the ganzfeld data has been volleyed back and forth just like the Ping-Pong balls that cover the subjects' eyes—so much so that Lisby decided she wanted to try it herself.

Submitting herself to the Ping-Pong ball/headset setup, Lisby volunteered to be a receiver while someone else tried to telepathically send her one of six images. When she was unhooked from the gizmo, she stared blankly at the six cards. Not a single one of them looked like anything that had popped into her mind during the experiment. The only thing she could muster up was "red." So when the grad student insisted she had to pick one image, even if it was just a random guess, Lisby picked the image with the red sunset.

The grad student opened the envelope to show Lisby which image had been transmitted to her. It was the red sunset.

Lisby writes, "At that moment, the world turned weird. I felt the tiniest instant of overwhelming fear. It was gone in a flash but it was stunningly real. It was unlike any fear I've ever felt. My mind split. I realized that I knew something I was simultaneously certain I didn't know. And I got it. This is what my patients meant when they said, 'My mind is not my own.' Or 'I'm losing my mind.' The feeling was terrifying. My mind had slipped out from under me and the world felt out of control . . . After I left the lab, I realized I'd gotten what I'd come for: some feeling for a quality of knowing that gave me that hook for believing . . . Part of me still insisted that picking the red sunset was merely coincidence, no more than a lucky guess and nothing to do with the ganzfeld state or tuning down the noise. But believing in the extraordinary tuning in wasn't what I came for. I'd come for something different. Not the jolt I'd felt when that graduate student handed me the sunset card, or when the young man gave me back the harp . . . The jolt was a signal after the fact. I'd come to find the feeling *before* the jolt . . . Whatever that sensation was, that's what I'd come for."

Is telepathy real? If so, does this prove that we are all One and that we are capable of somehow hooking into the field of consciousness that links us all? I can't say for sure, but the prospects are tantalizing. Regarding this topic, Lisby concludes, "As human beings, might we be capable of a connectedness with other people and every other aspect of our material world so profound that it breaks all the rules of nature as we know it? If so, it's a connectedness so radical as to be practically inconceivable."

RADICAL CONNECTION

If we really are connected at this level, what does it mean for the way we live together in our world? It's so easy to fall into judgment of those who don't believe or behave the way we do, but every time we sit in judgment of one another, we perpetuate the illusion of separation, forgetting the Oneness that unites us. We're all guilty of this. I recently posted an inspirational video on Facebook that shared the message of a famous spiritual teacher. Many were touched by the video and shared it with their friends, but a few wrote disparaging remarks, claiming that the spiritual teacher couldn't be trusted because he struggled with alcoholism, as if we could never trust anything we might learn about spirituality from an alcoholic.

I found myself reflecting back on the 12-step meetings I was required to sit in on as part of my psychiatry rotation during my medical training. Attending these meetings with active and recovering addicts touched me deeply. I had grown up judging addicts as lost souls who simply lacked willpower. I certainly never thought you could trust an addict with teaching you anything spiritual. But witnessing these meetings, I was humbled to realize that these individuals had much to teach me about what spirituality really means. I hadn't realized that, in my judgment, I was committing one of the greatest spiritual offenses. I had forgotten that compassion is perhaps the most spiritual of virtues, and compassion was what these Alcoholics Anonymous attendees had in spades.

As I listened to the addicts tell their stories of human vulnerability, heads nodded around the circle from others who understood. They told stories of childhood sexual abuse, parental abandonment, foster homes, and alcoholic parents. They had been beaten with golf clubs. Their mothers had knocked out their teeth. Some had been moved from orphanage to orphanage, being forced to leave the only people they found to love in each home.

They hadn't just been traumatized themselves. Some had become perpetrators of trauma. They confessed how they had hurt others—betraying those they loved, stealing money from their parents, breaking laws and even violently harming other humans. They spoke of blackouts and seizures, suicide attempts and jail time and the shame they felt about beating up their spouses and children. As they told their stories, often through tears, the others listened generously, often in tears themselves. Nobody judged these addicts as they told their stories. Instead, everyone listened with pure, loving compassion. It was downright holy. I found myself deeply moved as I communed in Oneness with my fellow human life travelers, and I felt ashamed of how I had judged them.

Every single one of us is doing the best we can. None of us have it all figured out, even the ones you might be tempted to put on a pedestal. Do any of us want to be judged for our mistakes when we're trying as hard as we can to be our best selves? The world doesn't need more judgment. We need more compassion. An anonymous quote that sums it all up says, "Don't judge someone just because they sin differently than you." When we make compassion a practice, we bless the world.

It's not just others who need our compassion; it's ourselves. So often, when we judge others, what we're really doing is projecting our own self-criticism onto another. When we judge another, we're often criticizing disavowed shadow parts of ourselves. If I get all righteous because I think I'm superior to someone, I can always find that, at least on some level, I am also the very thing I'm judging. For example, if I'm triggered by a friend because I feel she's being selfish, I need look no further than myself to find why I'm triggered by her behavior—because I, too, can be selfish. Because it's easier to criticize others than to examine our own shadows, we project our own unexamined shadow traits onto others, when we're better off practicing compassion with others and ourselves.

Judgment stems from false fear. We are afraid when others are different than we are. If someone worships a different deity or loves a same-sex partner or chooses to terminate a pregnancy or aligns with the opposite political party, we judge. When someone comes from a warring clan or an enemy gang or the other side of the tracks, we make them "other." When someone commits a crime, we judge. Yet every time we do this, we hurt ourselves. We're afraid of people who are different than we are, as if the fact that they're not exactly like us somehow threatens our own sense of self. But it is only the Small Self that is threatened. If we are willing to let fear heal us, we can use our fears to illuminate how our prejudices feed into the illusion of separation. When we can get our own Small Selves out of the way, we can experience others soul-to-soul, and differences dissolve. The soul is never threatened by such differences.

Our Small Selves feel safer if everyone conforms, but every individual is as unique as a snowflake. At the same time, we are also interconnected through a collective consciousness that unites us all. It's a paradox the cognitive mind simply can't understand. Even trying to think about it short-circuits the brain. As Jill Bolte Taylor experienced when she had a left brain stroke, only the right hemisphere can understand that we are all One. We can't reason our way to Oneness, because the minute we engage the reasoning left brain, it makes us separate. It says, "I am." And if "I am," then "You are," and with this dualistic worldview, we are no longer One.

The left hemisphere of the brain gets us into a lot of trouble, as individuals, as a species, and as citizens of our world. False fear originates in the left hemisphere of the brain, where language lives, because every false fear is nothing but a thought, a figment of language. Because the left hemisphere also creates this illusion of separation, distinguishing between "I am" and "You are," conflicts and traumas arise, and we are able to inflict all kinds of emotional and physical violence not only upon one another, but also upon our planet.

Most of the global challenges we face as citizens of earth arise from the mistaken notion that we are separate beings, disconnected from one another and from Source. The moment we remember that we are all One, we can no longer turn our backs on other suffering humans, endangered animals, the destruction of rainforests, polluted oceans, and a thinning atmosphere. If we are all One, we are only as strong as our weakest link, and our weakest links lie in the devastation of the natural world right now. At no other time in the history of our planet has one species been responsible for the total destruction of other planetary life. As long as we're stuck in the illusion of separation, we're capable of making selfish choices that might keep us more comfortable in the short term but in the long term, we will destroy the natural world, and with it, ourselves as a species.

When we remember that we are all One, we will be called to open our hearts to unprecedented levels of compassion. Rather than succumbing to fear, dividing ourselves with judgment, or throwing our hands up in helplessness, we will be called to action. The choice is ours.

How do we do this? Where do we start? It all begins with YOU. When even one person makes the choice to heal false fear and choose compassionate courage instead, this choice ripples out, infecting and entraining others with the love that accompanies it. Even one human walking around in the world with an unarmored heart, choosing right action from that place, blesses others. Radiating love, even in small ways, raises the vibration of the planet. When we remember who we really are, we remind others of their own true nature, and the illusion of separation begins to dissolve.

THE 51ST DEER

In Tom Shadyac's documentary film *I Am,* an animated cartoon points a finger at the insanity of our human selfishness. The cartoon tells the story of an indigenous tribe that lived in harmony for many years, nurturing and caring for one another, tending one another when anyone was hungry or sick. Then one day, the tribe's best hunter decided to start keeping what he killed for himself, hoarding his stash on a mountain far from the tribe. When the other star hunters saw what he was doing, they started hoarding their kills too, while those who were weaker and sicker were left hungry. As the tribe shifted to a culture of greed and competition, parents began teaching their children how to get more of the fruits of the hunt for themselves, transforming the tribe from a healthy, sustaining collective organism into a disconnected band of separate, self-absorbed individuals.

Sound familiar? Just look at the way the world is today. The illusion of separation drives a small percentage of the global population to hoard resources and pillage the environment at the expense of the health and well-being of most of humanity and the natural world. But it doesn't have to be this way. Nothing but fear is perpetuating this cycle. We're afraid our own needs or the needs of our families won't be met if we adopt a more cooperative mentality. We're afraid of political ideologies such as socialism because historical experiments with such philosophies have led us to associate socialism with dictatorship and the erosion of freedom. Yet these failed experiments were nothing but another example of the star hunter hoarding the meat.

As humans, we are the only species who lives in this competitive, dog-eat-dog manner. Perhaps we can learn something from other animals. Shadyac's film describes an experiment conducted with a herd of red deer to determine their true nature: Are they instinctually competitive or cooperative? For months, scientists monitored the herd in order to analyze how deer culture operates. Here's what they discovered.

Every day, when it was time to go drink from the watering hole, the deer engaged in a sort of voting ritual. The alpha deer didn't dictate which watering hole they would drink from and drag the unwilling with him. Instead, all the deer had the opportunity to point their heads toward the watering hole of their choice. When at least 51 percent of the deer chose the same watering hole, the majority ruled, and the rest would follow. When it came time to change watering holes, the same ritual applied.

The take-home message from the film *I Am* is that we're in the midst of a planetary shift in consciousness from one of greed and competition to one of cooperation and sustainability. Tom Shadyac said, "The solution begins with a deeper transformation that must occur in each of us. *I Am* isn't as much about what you can do, as who you can be. And from that transformation of being, action will naturally follow."

What would happen if 51 percent of the human race stopped letting false fear rule their lives? Let's find out. It all starts with you. You just might be the 51st deer that crosses the threshold and takes us past what Malcolm Gladwell calls "the tipping point." When you make this personal choice, you participate in healing the world. Margaret Mead said, "Never doubt that a small group of thoughtful, committed citizens can change the world; indeed, it's the only thing that ever has."

Perhaps 51 percent is all it takes to shift global consciousness. Perhaps it's also all you need in order to let fear free you, so your natural courage can emerge. In order to make the decisions in a corporation, you don't need to own 100 percent of the stock. All you need is 51 percent. When your soul buys out your Small Self and gains control of 51 percent of the stock in the company of YOU, courage takes charge.

Part Three of this book is all about getting you to your own personal 51 percent mark. In Part Three, you'll learn the Six Steps to Cultivating Courage and have the opportunity to write your own Prescription for Courage. By the end of the book, you'll have an intuitively created action plan for how to transform fear into fuel for growth so you can let courage take the wheel.

COURAGE-CULTIVATING EXERCISE #12

Tonglen Meditation for Compassion

Tonglen, a Tibetan Buddhist practice of taking on the suffering of others and replacing it with your happiness, compassion, and peace through your breath, has numerous benefits. It dissolves the self-protection, clinging, and fixation of the Small Self and opens the heart. It reverses the Small Self's tendency to avoid suffering and seek pleasure and liberates you from the prison of selfishness. In the beginning, you may find that you resist this practice. It may bring up all your revulsion, resentment, frustration, anger, and avoidance of suffering. If you experience these feelings, use them to deepen the practice. Let the poison of life's suffering become the medicine. By doing this practice, your heart will open more and more and you will become a vessel of compassion that heals others with your presence. Imagine a world in which we all practiced tonglen every day.

1. Start by cleansing your emotional landscape. Sit quietly and focus on your breath as you allow your mind to become still. Using your breath, see yourself breathing in any negative emotions you might be feeling right now, then breathing out peace and joy. Purify your emotional landscape by repeating this process until you feel calm and clear.

2. Next, cleanse yourself. See yourself as two beings— your Inner Pilot Light and your Small Self. As you breathe in, visualize your Inner Pilot Light breathing in all of your Small Self's suffering into its wide-open heart. As you breathe out, see your Inner Pilot Light sending your Small Self healing, peace, calm, love, and compassion. In the compassionate embrace of your Inner Pilot Light, your Small Self then responds by opening its heart too, and all of the suffering dissolves.

3. Cleanse your wrongdoings by considering a situation where you didn't behave as your best self. Maybe you feel guilty or ashamed or regretful. As you think about this situation, accept responsibility for this event as you breathe in, then as you breathe out, acknowledge your wrongdoing and send forgiveness to yourself and offerings of love, peace, and reconciliation to the ones you harmed.

4. Now that you've cleansed your emotional land-
    scape, your Small Self's pain, and moved into the
    energy of forgiveness and reconciliation, expand
    your tonglen practice for others. Start with just one
    person you want to help. Invoke the presence of
    the Divine in your heart, then as you feel the pain
    or suffering this person is feeling, visualize the pain
    as grimy black smoke that you breathe in. As you
    breathe it in, this toxic smoke dissolves in the open-
    ness of your heart and purifies your heart of any of
    the Small Self's grasping, self-protection, or self-
    absorption that prevents you from sensing the One-
    ness of all beings. As you breathe out, see yourself
    spreading light, love, compassion, and happiness to
    the one in pain.

5. Now expand this practice beyond one person into
    the collective. Breathe in the suffering of others,
    then as you breathe out, see the rays of this light,
    love, and compassion touching every soul on the
    planet. This practice can be very powerful, infusing
    the energy of compassion into the culture and con-
    necting us in our web of Oneness.

6. If you find yourself resisting this practice, notice any
    emotions that come up—resentment, fear, anger,
    sadness, terror, revulsion, feelings of revenge. Also
    notice any physical sensations—tightness in your
    chest, gripping in your solar plexus, or a feeling of
    heaviness or darkness. As you breathe in, feel the
    Oneness with all of the other people on the planet
    who are feeling just like you do. As you breathe
    out, send relief to all the suffering beings, including
    yourself.

COURAGE-CULTIVATING EXERCISE #13

Enemies and Heroes

The following exercise is adapted from an exercise Martha Beck teaches with me to health care providers at the Whole Health Medicine Institute, inspired by the work of Byron Katie.

- Think of someone who makes you absolutely crazy. Who really gets your goat? Who has wronged you? Who do you think deserves to rot in hell? Now write that person a letter. Start the letter with "Dear _____, In my darkest hours, here's what I really, truly think of you." Then let loose. Don't try to be enlightened. Let your Small Self have at it. Rip this person a new one. Really go for it. (And don't worry. Nobody but you has to read this letter.)

- Now think of someone you really admire. This person can be alive or dead. You don't even have to know this person. You can pick Jesus or Buddha if you like. But make sure it's someone you really love, who represents all the human qualities you most respect and appreciate. Write this person a letter that starts with "Dear _____, In my darkest hours, here's what I really, truly think of you." Then gush like crazy. Go wild with praise.

- For Step 3 of this exercise, you'll need to listen to the instructions you can download free at TheFearCureBook.com. (Trust me! There's a reason I'm making you take this extra step. You'll see why when you listen to the instructions of my voice guiding you through the next step.)

COURAGE-CULTIVATING EXERCISE #14

Oneness Meditation

Find a quiet spot to sit and relax. If it resonates with you, put on some quiet music. Sit comfortably, close your eyes, and allow yourself 20 minutes to reflect upon the experience of Oneness that unites us all. Allow any illusions of separation to arise in order to illuminate them. Notice where you are judging someone or focusing on your own well-being to the detriment of another. Allow yourself to examine any ways in which you choose your own comfort over the well-being of the planet. Allow golden light to shine upon what arises so it can be released down a grounding cord into the core of the earth. Instead, allow yourself a chance to meditate upon the interconnectedness you feel with all beings. Become One with all humans, even those with whom you struggle. Allow yourself to become One with all animals. Be One with all plant life, including the forests. Feel the Oneness with the ocean, the mountains, the meadows, the rivers, the lakes, the soil, and all of Mother Earth. Experience the Oneness with the moon, the sun, the planets, the stars, and all of the cosmos. Allow yourself to become a vessel for golden light as it flows through you and into the earth, grounding and connecting you to all beings through this earth grounding. Allow this light within you to extend out of the top of your head, connecting you to the cosmos, so that you become nothing but light transmitting up, down, and all around, connecting you in Oneness to All That Is.

To be led through a guided Oneness meditation, download the free Prescription for Courage Kit at TheFearCureBook.com.

PART THREE

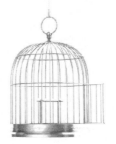

The
PRESCRIPTION
for **COURAGE**

CHAPTER 8

FREE YOURSELF

Courage is fear that has said its prayers.

— Dorothy Bernard

As Dennis and I waited in line to ride the biggest, scariest roller coaster in the amusement park, we only got glimpses of what was ahead for us. We couldn't see the whole roller coaster from where we waited, just enough to make us apprehensive about the uncertainty of what we were about to experience. As we moved forward in line, our stomachs filled with butterflies. We watched people board the coaster, then, a few minutes later, they'd un-strap themselves and exit the ride. Nobody seemed to be dying. We found this mildly reassuring, but a question remained—would we survive too?

Finally, we were strapped in, the safety bars locked, the roller coaster poised to jet forward, the unknown looming before us. There was no turning back. After accelerating from a dead stop to 60 miles per hour in a few seconds, leaving our stomachs far behind our bodies, the coaster rose, clackety-clacking up the first hill, slowly, our anticipation rising with each foot of elevation. Dennis and I looked into each other's eyes with one of those *What the hell were we thinking?* looks. We were both scared, but there was also the glimmer of excitement. What were we about to experience? I was grateful for the company. At least I wasn't venturing into the unknown alone.

Even from our front-row seat, we couldn't see what was over the crest of the hill. The track ahead dipped just low enough so you couldn't see where you were going. I noticed myself bracing. I recognized this feeling. It's how I often feel when I'm about to take a risk and try something out of my comfort zone. I felt it when I brought my newborn baby home. I felt it when I quit my job as a practicing physician. I felt it when I decided to end my marriage. I felt it when I confessed my love to someone I wasn't sure loved me back. I felt it when I decided to risk putting my first book out into the world. I still feel it every time I get up on stage to give a speech to thousands of people. During all of those situations, I noticed a tendency to brace against the uncertainty, the same way I was doing now as the roller coaster climbed.

I remembered a piece of art created by Brian Andreas that had reassured me as I prepared to quit my job: the figure of a woman sitting in an upside-down umbrella, inscribed with the words *If you hold on to the handle, she said, it's easier to maintain the illusion of control. But it's more fun if you just let the wind carry you.* It took me years to muster up the courage to quit my stable job, but these words helped. Reminding myself that it's more fun if you let go of the handle helped me stop bracing against the uncertainty so I could trust instead.

Just as the roller coaster roared over the top of the hill, I grabbed Dennis's hand and yelled over the noise of the machine, "Let go!" I tried to relax my belly just as my solar plexus gripped in the free fall. We both let go of the safety bar and raised our arms up in the air, our legs dangling like noodles, just as the coaster plunged toward the earth. Throughout the rest of the ride, I repeated the mantra to myself: *Let go let go let go . . .*

The coaster twisted upside down, flew through a loop, and tore us around a corner. At one point, we stopped at the top of a loop, the coaster holding us upside down in total stillness. Only the safety bar stood between us and the ground far below. Dennis yelled, "This is too scary!" as he gripped the safety bar, but he was laughing the whole time. If you're able to trust that you're safe, fear can be transformed into a thrill. Without trust, fear is just plain scary.

By the end of the ride, our stomach muscles were sore from uncontrollable laughter. Our bodies were shaking a bit from the rush of adrenaline. When we hobbled off the cart, dizzily stumbling like two drunk people, both of us said at the same time, "Again!" The second time wasn't nearly as scary. We knew what to expect, so we were able to relax more, surrender more, lean into the free fall and hang upside down without gripping so tightly. But it wasn't quite as exciting the second time around. The uncertainty of a roller coaster you don't know is more thrilling than one you've ridden a dozen times.

Life can be the same way. We can guard against uncertainty, resist what lies outside our comfort zone, and grip the safety bar when we feel afraid. Or we can use our discernment in order to choose to take appropriate risks, so life can be exciting, fun, and filled with meaning, purpose, and love. Cultivating courage is not about being reckless and rushing headlong into scary situations without suitable caution. It's also not about traumatizing yourself. A friend of mine is terrified of roller coasters, and a spiritual teacher she worked with required his students to ride roller coasters in order to learn to let go. She says it didn't help her at all. All that happened when she was forced to ride roller coasters is that her nervous system wound up on perpetual red alert. She had to learn to let go in her own way.

Most people don't cultivate courage by being thrust into scary situations against their will. You're better off stretching yourself than having someone else push you too hard. What does help is putting yourself in situations that stretch you beyond your comfort zone in the presence of others who help you feel safe. But you have to be ready. You must really want to let fear grow you so courage can blossom. Doing so is all about learning to trust that you are safe, connected, and always being guided toward your true nature and your life's purpose.

FEELING SAFE

At some point in your life, you may have experienced that sense of absolute safety that comes from trusting something or someone. Maybe you remember being a child, in the arms of your unconditionally loving grandmother, where you felt completely safe because Nana was in charge. Maybe your mother and father were always fighting; maybe Dad was an abusive alcoholic or Mom had psychiatric problems and was always exploding, so you learned to grip the controls of life because it wasn't safe at home any other way. If you weren't in control, always guarding against uncertainty, bad things happened. But with Nana, you knew you could just *let go.* When you did, the gripping in your belly relaxed and you felt free to be your playful, magical child self. Nana made you feel brave in a way nobody else did, so you were free to ride the biggest slide at the playground, the one that scared you when you were there with only Mom. You trusted that you didn't have to play it safe all the time when Nana was with you; she helped you cultivate the natural courage inside of you.

Or maybe you never experienced that feeling of trust and safety growing up, but you felt it when you fell in love. Because you trusted your beloved so completely, you were willing to take crazy risks, as long as your beloved was there beside you. You trusted something bigger than even that one beloved person. You trusted this thing called love so much that the gripping fear you may have felt before loosened, and you were willing to give up everything that once made you feel safe and in control. You didn't need to be in charge anymore, because your lover was with you, and the love you shared made you brave.

You can't open your soul cage by yourself. It requires sharing great trust with another to unlock the prison that keeps the soul safe. While this is true, the problem with this kind of courage is that it depends upon another human being, and inevitably, other humans will fail us. Perhaps Nana died, and you felt like you lost your courage when you lost her. Maybe your lover left you, and your fears came rearing up, leaving you feeling completely unsafe in a dangerous world all over again. If we're always seeking our safety in our relationships, if what we trust is other people, we're going to keep collecting evidence that it's not really safe to trust, because people are always at risk of letting us down. Even the most faithful, loyal, and unconditionally loving human may one day die before we do and leave us.

To cultivate courage in a sustainable, healthy way, we must begin to trust in something more. Perhaps you sense this thing you trust outside yourself, and call it God or Buddha or Allah or Mother Gaia. Perhaps you don't sense it outside, but within, where you trust your highest self—the voice of your Inner Pilot Light. If you don't believe in a guiding force—whatever its origin—that helps you stay aligned with your purpose, the cognitive mind feels like it has to stay in control and keep a tight grip on the safety bar. It won't loosen its grip until it has evidence that it's safe to let go. While surrounding ourselves with others who can help us is a necessary part of any real transformation, real lasting courage stems from trusting something more steadfast and reliable than any human being.

Perhaps you've already had an experience that has given you at least a taste of this feeling of ultimate safety, when you knew you were held in the arms of the unconditional love of something Divine. Maybe, like the people Lisby interviewed, you've known something you shouldn't have known, and this experience of anomalous cognition offered you evidence that there may be something beyond the physical plane that is always guiding and protecting you. Maybe you believe you've been visited by an angel or the spirit of someone you love who died, and this visitation gave you personal evidence that there might be something more that you could trust. Perhaps you've had a near-death experience, and you were so filled with certainty that death merges you into pure unconditional love that you were no longer afraid to die, and this granted you courage. Maybe you've experienced a "kundalini awakening" like the kind described by the yogic tradition. Maybe you've had a spontaneous mystical experience while in nature when you felt a Oneness with all beings. Maybe you've had a physical healing through nontraditional modalities, such as a visit to John of God or an experience with an energy medicine practitioner or an indigenous healer. Maybe you've had a left brain stroke like Jill Bolte Taylor and personally experienced the state of fearlessness that accompanies freedom from the cognitive mind. Maybe you've been on a shamanic journey that opened you to a realm beyond the limitations of our purely physical world. Maybe, like Lisby, you've had your own "This changes everything" experience, and it's offered concrete evidence to your cognitive mind that life is not to be feared; it's meant to be embraced with joy. Maybe your cognitive mind isn't as dense as people like me, and you haven't needed any evidence at all because you simply have blind faith in the Divine—and that's enough for you to trust and let go.

THE SHIFT TO PEACE

Each of us is unique, so the process of cultivating courage is going to be different for each of us, but the first step lies in being willing to at least entertain the idea that there's something bigger that you can trust to guide your life. As long as you don't trust anything other than your cognitive mind, you're likely to feel frightened. Your mind doesn't think it's safe to let go, and you want to micromanage every detail of your life. Then when life doesn't go as planned, you feel even more afraid, and you try even harder to control life. Uncertainty becomes something to be avoided at all costs. The idea of loss becomes intolerable. It seems like a dangerous world, and you wind up feeling all alone.

Once you take the leap of faith that allows you to turn over even a small bit of control to this thing you begin to trust, you'll start collecting evidence to prove to the cognitive mind that it really is safe to step into the unknown. As it starts getting proof that it's safe, the cognitive mind relaxes, fear lessens, and something inside of you begins to open up. The cognitive mind becomes a willing servant, rather than a brutal master, and the Small Self reluctantly takes its rightful position in the backseat. Then, because you become brave enough to let fear grow you, you begin to let courage take the lead in your life, rather than being at fear's mercy.

It's important to understand that making this shift doesn't eliminate fear. It would be unrealistic to think that you'd never have a false fear thought ever again, that if you learn to trust and let go, you'll be 100 percent fear-free. The reality is that you're still likely to hear the voice of your Small Self, prattling on, but you no longer need to allow this part of you to make your decisions, because on some higher level, you trust that you're safe. Freed from identification with your Small Self, you're able to tap into the wisdom and discernment of your Inner Pilot Light so you can muster up the moxie to do what you must, even when what you must do isn't exactly what you desire. Even when it scares you.

When fear does pop up (and it will), you don't automatically react to it. Instead, you question it. With open curiosity, you ask what it's trying to teach you. You explore the edges of your growth. You allow fear to be a marker for your progress. As time goes on, fear lessens. You feel more serene, and the space between fearful thoughts stretches out. This inner spaciousness and peace signals that you're making progress on the path to cultivating courage.

How does this shift happen? Transforming from unconsciously letting fear make your decisions to letting courage take the lead is an inside job. There's nothing anyone else can do to make this shift for you. You can certainly be proactive about facilitating this process. You can practice the tools shared in this book. You can consult with psychologists and doctors. You can seek out the guidance of spiritual advisors or go to your place of worship. You can read as many self-help books and spiritual texts as you like. You can take workshops and go on meditation retreats and follow the well-worn paths of spiritual seekers who have sought similar shifts. But ultimately, the shift happens internally, in its own perfect way, on its own time schedule. You can't force it, no matter how much your Small Self grabs hold of the desire to cultivate courage and tries to effort its way to success. Cultivating this kind of courage is not about doing more, it's about letting go, and nobody can let go for you. You'll have to guide this process of letting go yourself. That's what writing your own Prescription for Courage is all about. What I'll share in this part of the book will give you a framework to guide you through the process, but you'll have to fill in the frame yourself.

Keep in mind that you are not a helpless victim of your fear. Instead, be grateful for all fear is here to teach you. Fear is not something to resist; it's there to pinpoint where more trust is needed so you can lean into peace and find your brave. In the spirit of full transparency, let me warn you that while moving toward peace might sound gentle and easy, your Small Self will pull out all the stops to make it a rough road.

The process of letting fear free you and letting courage take charge is not for the faint of heart. You're going to be asked to face the truth about who you are and who you're not. The process requires complete honesty and radical self-compassion as you pierce the façade of untruth the Small Self has created, ostensibly to "protect" you. During this process of discovery and development, you'll be asked to come face-to-face with everything you imagined to be true, so you can put everything up for question. In doing so, you'll bring to light all that hides in the shadows. You'll have to stop denying what is true for you, even if it's scary to face the truth.

Most of us are so blinded by self-deception, so hooked into the fearful lies of our Small Self, that we don't even know what's true anymore. We may sense the truth, but it's often uncomfortable to face it head-on. The truth can be both brutal and wonderful: it requires examining all the limiting beliefs that are operating our lives unconsciously, and when we realize how we're creating our own suffering, it can be painful. Your fear may even rear up before it quiets down, because once you take the blinders off and illuminate all that is untrue in your life, you'll be more conscious of how false fear may be ruling your life. This realization may be supremely uncomfortable. But remember, any fear that gets unearthed is just more fodder for growth. Don't get frustrated; just keep returning to gratitude.

The truth may require you to admit that you're unhappy in a committed relationship. You may have to face the fact that you're selling your soul or your self-care for a paycheck. You may have to set boundaries with an abusive family member, and this may require distancing yourself from a relationship that really matters to you. You may have to learn to say no when others are used to your agreeable, people-pleasing Small Self. This may not go over so well with those you care about. That's why courage is necessary. Making choices that align with your soul's integrity isn't easy.

So why bother? Why put yourself at risk of so much discomfort? Why not leave fear in the shadows where it belongs? Because fear is the gateway to freedom. Once the fear is illuminated, it's cause for celebration. Now you know what lies between you and serenity. Yeah!

Martha Beck suggests that we're here on earth to mine emotion, including the emotion of fear. Just like it's more fun to ride a roller coaster you've never ridden before, life is more fun if we get to experience the full range of human emotion. Every emotion is here to help you move in the direction of peace. Cultivating courage isn't about rejecting fear; it's about transforming it into an opportunity for soul growth. Beyond the fear lies the place that feels like coming home. Courage arises from this place of peace.

When you're brave enough to write your Prescription for Courage and take action upon your inner guidance, you'll start to recognize right away why it's worth the effort. When you realize you live in a purposeful universe that is always guiding you to come into alignment with who you really are, you start to trust something you may not have trusted before, and this trust makes you brave. Over time, you lose interest in trying to force things to happen the way you once did. You become more interested in *letting* things happen the way they're meant to. Anxiety lessens. Unmet longing is unburdened from your heart. You fear less. You trust more.

Then magic begins to happen in ways you couldn't have anticipated. Once you embark upon the journey to cultivate courage, whatever Universal Intelligence guides and supports you does a little happy dance because you're finally on your way to peeling back all the layers of what isn't the *real you* in order to become who you really are. All that isn't you falls away. All that is you radiates.

WHO WOULD YOU BE IF FEAR WASN'T STOPPING YOU?

What would you do if you weren't afraid? What leaps of faith might you take? How might you love? What kinds of relationships might you have? What kind of work might you do? How might you serve others? What truth would you speak? What aspects of the real you would you unveil? How would you live if every aspect of your life aligned with the values of your soul? How would you feel if nothing was holding you back from living your bravest life?

Imagine this. Instead of waking up afraid of what the day holds, you open your eyes feeling excited about the possibilities that lie ahead of you. You notice yourself focusing less on what you lack and more on what you appreciate. When negative emotions naturally arise, you move quickly through feelings of fear, anxiety, depression, disappointment, resentment, anger, and frustration into feelings of peace, stillness, and joy. You no longer feel you have to compromise your integrity in order to get what you want. You discover greater meaning and purpose in your work. You prioritize relationships with others who are seeking to live beyond the grip of fear, so you can support each other in your desire to live more courageously. Your heart becomes less guarded. The sense of disconnection, loneliness, and separation that may have plagued you gets replaced by openhearted feelings of love, compassion, and connection with all beings. You discover an upwelling of enthusiasm for dreams, activities, and passions you've suppressed. Instead of defending against loss, you accept it as an inevitable process of initiation that grows your soul. Rather than feeling threatened by that which you don't know or understand, you are simply curious. The Small Self who once chattered away in your mind, frightening you with artificial doom and gloom, quiets down. You sense, instead, an inner stillness that offers you refuge and makes you brave. Your newfound courage doesn't lead you to behave recklessly, because you are guided by your integrity. Steered by your inner compass, you have no need to let false fear drive your decisions and actions.

Once you make this shift, you may notice some surprising side effects. Others are magnetized to your kindness and inner calm, and you may discover that you're drawing to you people who tune to a whole different vibration. This inner peace may also spill into your professional life, helping you close the deal, attracting clients, fueling new ideas, and generating more revenue. You may notice that you become a wellspring of unexpected creativity, since fear limits creativity, while your intuition is creativity's best muse. Your sex life may heat up because you're no longer afraid to unleash your most authentic sexual self. Your physical appearance may change, and others may comment on how much more beautiful you appear when your inner light shines more on the outside. You may notice that your body feels more energetic, you more easily maintain a healthy weight, and physical symptoms that may have plagued you clear up. In some instances, you may even be surprised to find that chronic illnesses spontaneously resolve without medical treatment. If fear isn't ruling your decisions, your whole life can change.

LET YOUR INNER PILOT LIGHT TAKE THE LEAD

Rachel Naomi Remen recently told me that when she met me in 2007, there was a part of me she recognized right away, even though we had never met—a part that was authentic and wise. She explained to me that the part of me she recognized only had about 20 percent stock in what she called "the company of Lissa." She became curious about whether this 20 percent part would ever take charge. She suspected it would as I matured.

In 2013, we started teaching together and spending a lot of time together personally. Rachel said of that time, "I realized that the part of you I recognized when we met—the old, wise Lissa— finally had about 48 percent stock in the company of Lissa." She reminded me that, in order to run a company, you don't need to own 100 percent of the stock; you only need 51 percent in order to have the deciding vote in all of the company decisions. Rachel sensed that the older, wiser part of me—the part I call my Inner

Pilot Light—was gaining ground. Just as it only took 51 percent of the deer to guide the herd to a new watering hole, if 51 percent of you gets control of *you,* it can take the lead. If you stop letting your Small Self's fears direct all your decisions, courage is free to make your decisions instead. Rachel began advising me at that point, and much of what I learned from her is shared in this book.

I don't know that I've quite hit the 51 percent mark yet in my own personal and spiritual development. And I won't make any blind promises to you as we move into the last and most prescriptive chapter of this book. What I can promise you is that my intention is to fortify you to cultivate courage for yourself in the way only you can prescribe. In my own life, I'm still committed to this process, and I'm still working on my own Prescription for Courage to guide me toward the stillness and wisdom inside of me. (You can read my own ever-evolving Prescription for Courage in Appendix D.) I'm hoping that you will find within you the desire to seek the same for yourself in your own unique way.

When your Inner Pilot Light takes over 51 percent of you, something curious happens. It doesn't seize control and start forcing its way. It simply lets go of needing to always be in control and starts to trust something large and purposeful. The cognitive mind, dominated by the Small Self, has a hard time letting go as long as it thinks nobody it can trust is in control, but if you can trust that it's safe for your Inner Pilot Light to take the lead, you can calm this smaller part of you and help it let go. Letting go feels completely unnatural when you're afraid. It's so much more tempting to grasp in desperation and try to control your life. Yet letting your Inner Pilot Light take the lead requires trusting that it's safe to surrender control completely.

A part of you already recognizes that it's time to let go, that grasping at what you desire isn't working. Yet even the desire to let go can become its own form of grasping. The Small Self wants to figure out how to let go so it can do a good job controlling the process of letting go. The Small Self can grasp at this just as desperately as it grasps at achievement or romantic love. But it's not your job to control the process of letting go. All that you need to do is let things be exactly as they are. Don't judge yourself for feeling fearful. Just accept that you're afraid and let it be. Don't resist the pain you feel as the result of heartbreak or disappointment. Just be with heartbreak and disappointment. Don't cling to what you desire. Just accept the discomfort of your unmet longing. Remember the mantra "I accept. I accept. I accept." And let go of everything in you that's arguing with reality and trying to make the world different than it is.

Your Small Self will go ballistic if you tell it to let go. It will make up all kinds of stories about how dangerous it would be to simply accept what is. It will make up a script that berates you for being lazy or irresponsible or unrealistic. Yet your Inner Pilot Light knows that letting go isn't about shirking responsibility or ignoring your commitments or betraying your integrity. Letting go simply means being fully present with exactly what is in the present moment, without either resisting it or clinging to it because you're afraid to lose it. It means stepping into the part of you that is pure consciousness, completely accepting of everything exactly as it is.

This is part of what attracts us to nature. Nature isn't trying to change anything. It just is. Daffodil bulbs bloom as the snow melts without grasping at winter or resisting spring. The river flows around the rocks without getting mad at the rocks. The sun sets in a bloom of golden rose clouds without being disappointed that the day is over. Mountains aren't trying to be beautiful; they just are. Waves don't struggle to keep crashing on the beach; they just do. Redwood trees don't have to push themselves to radiate peace. Nature *just is.*

It's so very hard for us in our modern culture to let go. We have our ideas about how things are supposed to be, and whenever reality splits from what we think should happen, we get upset. We resist. We make reality wrong. We suffer. Nature has something to teach us when it comes to letting go. Just going outside and witnessing how nature operates can teach us much about how to live and let go.

Pain is inevitable, but suffering is optional. We can't avoid the pain of life. Tragedies will happen. We will lose people we love. We will have unmet desires. We will get sick and die. Such things are unavoidable, even when we take all precautions to avoid being reckless and protect ourselves from danger. As hard as it is for us to accept, we ultimately have no control over life's tragedies. Peace comes when we just accept whatever happens. It's possible to experience a strange sort of peace even in the moments when everything is unraveling. It's not about skipping the emotions of grief, loss, disappointment, anger, or sadness. It's about moving through them without resistance. What you'll find is that when you let yourself feel what you feel in the present moment without fearing it or making it wrong, peace is accessible always.

Letting go is the opposite of struggle. You don't have to try too hard to transform your relationship with fear and unearth your natural courage. In fact, the energy of struggle gets in the way. Letting go happens most effectively when you simply accept what is and lean into peace. The energy of peace and surrender draws to you the very things you desire. As Tosha Silver says, "The very act of grasping for the feather creates the wind current that pushes it away." Letting go isn't about giving up. It's just about giving up the grasping.

Writing your own Prescription for Courage requires letting go of the grasping, including grasping at the desire to cultivate courage. If you're too attached, you actually inhibit the process. It's all about *allowing* the process instead, from a place of ease and peace. What will it take to bring yourself closer to peace? What limiting beliefs might you need to illuminate and heal? Who might you need to surround yourself with in order to feel safe letting go? What might help you better hear the voice of your Inner Pilot Light, so you can strap your Small Self lovingly into the backseat and let your Inner Pilot Light take the wheel? What stands in the way between you and peace? How can you let that go? These are the kinds of questions you'll be asked to address in the next chapter.

In it, I'll be sharing with you the Six Steps to Cultivating Courage. This is not a tried-and-true formula you get to just follow blindly, nor a one-two-three process that allows you to abdicate responsibility for your own journey. It simply provides a framework in which you can allow your intuition to guide you, since as I've said, cultivating courage is an inside job.

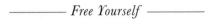

Keep in mind that this process is about doing less, not adding more to your "to do" list. As Lao Tzu wrote, "In the pursuit of knowledge, every day something is added. In the pursuit of enlightenment, every day something is dropped." The next chapter will assist you in determining what you need to drop so you can free yourself.

CHAPTER 9

SIX STEPS *to* CULTIVATING COURAGE

Your time is limited, so don't waste it living someone else's life.
Don't be trapped by dogma—which is living with the results of
other people's thinking. Don't let the noise of others' opinions
drown out your own inner voice. And most important, have the
courage to follow your heart and intuition.

— STEVE JOBS

Dennis and I were perched hundreds of yards up in the air on a wooden platform in a tree. Dennis was afraid of heights, so even though we were strapped in with harnesses we were assured would hold the weight of an elephant, his heart was pounding. The first obstacle in the black diamond ropes course, the most difficult of the four courses, required us to strap into a zip line that transported us from one treetop to another over a vast expanse of empty space, held in with a harness but with no safety net underneath. Next, we walked across a log that rocked between two wires. Further challenges along the course included balancing on top of vertical logs that hung like wind chimes, walking with our feet teetering in a series of black rings, and shuffling along a tight wire. If we were to fall, our guides promised us the harnesses would catch us, so our rational minds knew we were completely safe. But the moment you put your foot onto something wobbly when you're that high up in the trees, something primal takes over.

As Dennis approached the most difficult obstacle of the course, I watched him stand on the edge of the platform looking grim. He stared down at the ground below and said to me, "You go first." I started to move the lobster claws of my harness in front of his, but then he changed his mind. "It's less scary if you go first, but it's more fun if I do." He closed his eyes and took a moment to find his center internally, then he plunged into the obstacle, feeling the fear and doing it anyway. I cheered.

Dennis and I weren't riding roller coasters and dangling from ropes courses to traumatize ourselves. We chose to do these things as part of our own Prescriptions for Courage, pushing ourselves into uncomfortable situations in order to help ourselves let go.

Sometimes that's what it takes to let fear cure you. If you're brave enough to move gently and tenderly into your fear, you may find it loosening its grip on you, and slowly, like a seed sprouting, courage pushes through. Jia Jiang, whom I mentioned in Chapter 4, did the same thing regarding his fear of rejection. Jia had some painful experiences of rejection, but he recognized how fear of rejection was keeping him from fully living. In order to overcome this fear, he challenged himself to "100 Days of Rejection," during which he set out to make 100 crazy requests he assumed would be met with a no, as a way to desensitize himself through repetitive exposure. He asked strangers if he could borrow $100, play soccer in their backyard, be a live mannequin at Abercrombie & Fitch, sit in a police car's driver's seat. He asked for a private jet ride from Tony Hsieh and an interview with President Obama. He even asked a Krispy Kreme employee if she could make a special Olympic-symbol donut, and requested a "burger refill." Jia made videos of his requests and garnered an unexpected following of people who were rooting for him to overcome his fear of rejection. Surprisingly, many of his requests were granted, inspiring him with new respect for the kindness of strangers. But sometimes, he was rejected, and over time, rejection got easier. After challenging himself and surviving rejection, Jia said, "Our imagination often takes us to the worst possible outcome, causing us to be much less likely to take that action. We are really our own worst rejectors."

When I started blogging in 2009, one of my biggest fears was being perceived as imperfect. Growing up, I was the Goody Two-shoes who made straight A's, didn't drink, smoke, or use drugs, and was saving myself for marriage. As a doctor, I felt a great deal of pressure to be perfect in the hospital; otherwise, innocent people might die. I had started withholding the truth about who I really was or even telling little white lies to paint a picture of myself that was more "perfect" than I really was, and it left me feeling isolated, lonely, and hypocritical, as people tended to believe the picture, to think I was more perfect than I really was. I lived in constant fear of being "found out," and the shame of the lie I was living paralyzed me and damaged my relationships.

My intention with my blog was to be what I called "unapologetically ME" and to do so publicly. I used my blog as an opportunity to share with strangers how I was struggling with my own imperfections in my quest to be the most authentically Lissa I could be. I wanted to avoid my past tendency to gloss over the truth, take off the masks that protected me, practice being more vulnerable, and learn to deal with criticism. As it did for Jia, public accountability helped me stay true to my mission. I blogged very candidly about my fear of quitting my job, my failure to publish my first book, my painful realizations about how my ego operates, my marital struggles, my heartbreak in other relationships, my financial challenges, the mystical experiences that were unfolding as I walked my spiritual path, and other vulnerabilities I might have kept to myself in the past. In addition to desensitizing myself to my fear of being perceived as imperfect, I learned that most people didn't judge me or criticize me when I shared with them what was true for me. In fact, it was just the opposite. It's almost as if my blog community made a group agreement not to use my vulnerability against me. Brené Brown teaches that vulnerability is the gateway to intimacy and connection, and in my personal experience, this has proved to be true. My willingness to go public with my imperfections actually helped people trust me. Instead of positioning myself as a perfect doctor on a pedestal buttoned up in a starched white coat, I allowed myself to be perceived as human, and instead of damaging my reputation or leaving people judging me, this seemed to grant people a portal to connection with me that engendered even more trust. From this place of trust, I've been able to take people along on my own journey so that those of us cultivating courage together all feel less alone, including me. This sense of safe, soulful community fueled me to make difficult decisions some people might consider brave.

Over time, my Prescription for Courage shifted from publicly airing my dirty laundry on the Internet to diving into my own deepest shadows, either privately or in the discerning company of my therapists, spiritual advisors, and most trusted friends. This is where the real cultivation of courage arose. Publicly sharing my imperfections was scary enough, but it also became a crutch that fed my Small Self. Telling my story publicly fed my desire for approval, since I attracted many cheerleaders who praised me and helped externally validate the sometimes painful decisions I was making. But my Inner Pilot Light didn't want me to be either dependent on anyone else's approval or at risk of influence from anyone else's criticism. I needed to find peace within myself when I was diving into the real truth of my own self-deception, and this peace needed to come from deep inside the scary silence of me. The real stretch came when I pushed myself to simply sit still in meditation with my truth, which was scarier for me than any public confession of imperfection, more terrifying than winding up $200,000 in debt, and more destabilizing to my psyche than quitting my job as a doctor. Facing the demons inside my own mind pushed me further beyond my comfort zone than anything else I had ever done. Digging deep into the shadow parts of my Small Self got easier when I met Dennis, who was also bravely diving into the depths of his own self-deception on the road to his true self. While cultivating courage is ultimately an inside job, if even one other person travels beside you on your journey as an accountability partner, it's not quite so scary.

Your Prescription for Courage may not include roller coasters, ropes courses, rejection therapy, silent meditation, or baring your soul on the Internet. Your journey will be your own, guided by the wisdom of your Inner Pilot Light. Cultivating courage is not necessarily about forcing yourself to do things that terrify you, and this process is not meant to traumatize you. It's meant to sink you into peace, which is where you'll find your courage. You'll have your own way of letting fear nudge you into soul growth as you surrender into peace, and that's what this chapter can help you figure out.

HOW TO GET STARTED

Cultivating courage doesn't lend itself to a simple step-by-step process the way making Jell-O does. Every journey is as individual as a fingerprint. However, some aspects of the process are similar for almost everyone, and some practices are predictably helpful, such as finding the support of a professional who can guide you and finding your stillness through some form of daily practice. If you read my book *Mind Over Medicine,* the Six Steps to Cultivating Courage might look familiar, because the steps are parallel to the Six Steps to Healing Yourself that I laid out in that book. Because the process of cultivating courage is a journey of healing and transformation, the same six steps that work for healing the body can guide you as you cultivate courage.

That said, unlike the processes taught in many self-help books, this is not a one-size-fits-all cure. I'll be offering you tools and helping you brainstorm ideas, but many of these have been filtered through my own biases, beliefs, and personal preferences. Yours may be radically different, which is why nobody can write this prescription for you. As you read on, take ownership of this process. Borrow what resonates. Leave what doesn't. Get inspired. Let yourself imagine a life characterized by peace. What will it take for you to free yourself?

Six Steps to Cultivating Courage

Step 1: BELIEVE. Replace fear-inducing beliefs with courage-enhancing trust.

Step 2: SUPPORT. Seek out support from people around you—and offer your support to others.

Step 3: INTUITION. Learn to trust your intuition in order to discern true fear from false fear.

Step 4: DIAGNOSE. Identify what lies at the root of your false fear.

Step 5: PRESCRIBE. Write The Prescription for Courage for yourself.

Step 6: SURRENDER. Release attachment to outcomes and accept what is.

STEP 1: BELIEVE. *Replace fear-inducing beliefs with courage-enhancing trust.*

We saw in Part One how the body's stress responses can harm us—and how it's not just the responses to present, urgent stressors; it's the thoughts, beliefs, and stories we make up in our minds that trigger one stress response after another, which can harm us even more than the original stressors themselves. Stress is just fear in disguise, so what's the solution? We must cultivate beliefs that limit our stress responses and allow the mind to relax. You may not realize that most of your false fear stems from limiting beliefs you hold as truth. You may not even recognize that you carry these beliefs with you as baggage, because you've accepted them as such truth that you don't even question them.

For example, you may think that you'll only make money if you struggle and work really hard. Yet this is a limiting belief, not a hard-and-fast truth. Some people get paid to do what they love, and it doesn't feel like work at all. The false fear that may arise from such a belief is the fear that shifting toward a career that pays you to do what you love will leave you broke. Yet many brave people who have taken risks make abundant incomes doing what they love. As long as you're stuck in the limiting belief that you have to sacrifice and struggle in order to be financially secure, you'll never be able to make brave choices about your career.

You may also believe that romantic relationships always lose the spark, and it's normal to feel disconnected, bored, or lonely in a long-term relationship. Yet the truth is that some couples are still madly in love and passionately attracted to each other decades later. If you stick to this limiting belief, the false fear that may arise is that you may be afraid to ask your partner to work on the relationship with a therapist if you no longer feel connected to your partner. And if your partner isn't game to do the hard work of reigniting your intimate connection, you may be afraid to end the relationship because of other limiting beliefs, such as *The children will be destroyed if I get divorced,* or *Everyone will think I'm a bad person if I end my marriage,* or *I'll never find love again at my age.*

The Four Fearful Assumptions tend to be the overarching beliefs under which most other fear-inducing limiting beliefs fall. For example, the limiting belief that you have to struggle in order to make money might fall under "It's a dangerous world" and "Uncertainty is unsafe," while the belief that all relationships lose their passion and you have to just settle might fall under both "Uncertainty is unsafe" and "I can't handle losing what I cherish." Practicing the exercises in Part Two of this book can help you shift your beliefs so you can replace the Four Fearful Assumptions with the Four Courage-Cultivating Truths. This relaxes the mind, reduces stress responses, and can actually counterbalance the nervous system even in the midst of the most stressful of life's events. If you know that uncertainty is the gateway to possibility, then you're more likely to take a risk in your career or put your relationship at risk by asking your partner to work on it with you. If you trust that it's a purposeful universe, you won't be afraid even if you wind up in debt or your relationship ends because of the risks you took. Instead, you'll trust that even outcomes you didn't desire have purpose and that your soul is growing. You sense that it will all make sense at some point, and the risks will have been worth it, even if things didn't work out the way you planned.

While fear can be a vehicle for growth, shifting your beliefs so you feel less fear only makes your transformation easier. Therefore, the first step in the Six Steps to Cultivating Courage is to replace fear-inducing beliefs with courage-enhancing ones. We have to be careful about the beliefs we put into our minds about our relationship to life's stressors and the fears that can accompany them. Our nervous systems calm down when we can come into right relationship with uncertainty, make peace with loss, trust that we live in a purposeful universe, and remember that we are never alone. For most of us, these beliefs hide in the subconscious mind, where they run programs we learned in childhood without our awareness. We may not even realize we're operating on programs run by beliefs like *Look out for number one* or *Protect your heart at all costs.*

What limiting beliefs may be operating you? Part Two may have helped you become aware of some large-scale limiting beliefs that run your life. But you may have other beliefs that are playing out as patterns in your life. A surefire way to pinpoint where you might be unconsciously operating from fear-based limiting beliefs is to take a look at these repeating patterns. Perhaps you've married three alcoholics, you've been fired from every job you loved, you keep winding up with no money, or you get physical symptoms every time things seem to be going your way. When these things have happened, you may have made up stories that you were simply the victim of other people or bad luck. But chances are good that if something keeps happening over and over, a limiting belief underlies your misfortune.

Here are a few examples of limiting beliefs that might be predisposing you to outcomes you'd prefer to avoid, but you'll have a chance to consider your own.

NEGATIVE OUTCOME	LIMITING BELIEF
Dating abusive narcissists	I have to please others and sacrifice my own needs and well-being in order to earn love.
Repetitive financial struggles	Kind, loving, generous people don't accumulate money.
Multiple chronic illnesses	I have to give until I'm depleted in order to be worthy.
Consistent overachieving that fails to bring fulfillment	Nobody will love me unless I keep achieving more.
Insatiable desire to accumulate wealth	I won't survive unless my bank account is padded.
Chronic obesity in spite of a healthy diet	I'm not safe unless I'm protected from unwanted attention with extra weight.

COURAGE-CULTIVATING EXERCISE #15

Identify Your Patterns

1. Are there any negative patterns that keep repeating themselves in your life? List them. Be careful not to judge yourself. Practice self-compassion as you examine this question.

2. Does anyone in your family have either similar patterns or polar opposite patterns? Be careful not to judge these family members. Practice compassion with them too.

3. Can you identify any beliefs that might underlie such patterns? Often, you may have unknowingly inherited these beliefs from your parents, as they may have inherited these beliefs from theirs. This exercise is not about blaming your ancestors; it's about raising awareness of the limiting beliefs that may be operating you so you can illuminate them and heal them.

4.   If you identify any limiting beliefs, bring these up
     with a skilled therapist or coach, or investigate tech-
     niques for healing limiting beliefs and cementing
     new ones. For 13 tips on how to shift your beliefs,
     see Appendix A.

Optimism Versus Pessimism

Are you an optimist or a pessimist by nature? Because of how
they explain negative events to themselves, pessimists may find
it much harder to take courageous risks, while optimists find it
easier to be brave because they tend to believe things will work
out well, even when they're faced with challenges. Pessimists are
predisposed to believe that when bad things happen, it's personal, pervasive, and permanent. In other words, negative outcomes
result from their own failure ("It's all my fault"), apply not just
to this specific outcome, but to all outcomes ("I have bad luck
with everything"), and last indefinitely ("I'm never going to get a
break"). Good events, on the other hand, they believe to be just
the opposite. Positive outcomes are perceived to be temporary
("I just got lucky this time"), specific ("My luck only applies to
this one thing"), and impersonal ("It's not because of anything
I did"). Optimists are a whole different breed. They perceive bad
events to be temporary, specific, and external, while they believe
good events are permanent, pervasive, and stemming from their
own competence.

If pessimistic beliefs are keeping you from your natural courage, take comfort in the fact that optimism, like courage itself, is
something you can cultivate. In his book *Learned Optimism*, Martin
Seligman, Ph.D., teaches an exercise he calls the "ABC's"—an acronym for Adversity, Belief, and Consequences. When you encounter
adversity (A), the event becomes a thought, which is quickly translated into a belief (B). These beliefs then affect how you behave,
resulting in consequences (C). By learning to modulate how you
translate adversity into belief, you can affect the consequences that

arise in the aftermath of an adverse event. When you change your explanatory style, you can convert pessimistic thoughts into optimistic ones, and this can give you more courage.

For example, your boss yells at you at work (adversity). You get upset and think, *My boss is so ungrateful. She doesn't appreciate me. I never get recognition for my hard work* (belief). You then snap at your boss and turn in your report late, out of spite (consequences). Or your new boyfriend cancels a date you've been excited about (adversity). You tell yourself, *I knew he was too good to be true. He doesn't really care about me* (belief). You feel hurt, disappointed, angry, and depressed all day (consequences).

How can you change the beliefs that arise in the wake of adversity? For example, when your boss gets upset, instead of taking it personally, assuming it's permanent, and making it pervasive, tell yourself it's specific to this circumstance, temporary, and not about you. Instead of believing your boss doesn't appreciate you, you can be curious about whether your boss had a rough morning at home and you got inadvertently caught in the cross fire. Instead of taking passive-aggressive action, you can choose to respond with compassion. Even if your boss doesn't notice, you'll feel better, and because you'll feel braver, you might even feel able to confront your boss in a kind manner and initiate a tough conversation. Instead of assuming your boyfriend doesn't care about you and getting depressed, you can be curious about whether your boyfriend is just busy or needs some space. Find something else fun to do that night in order to lift your spirits.

COURAGE-CULTIVATING EXERCISE #16

Convert from Pessimism to Optimism

Martin Seligman, Ph.D., author of *Learned Optimism*, recommends keeping an ABC diary for a few days to assess the beliefs that arise in the face of adverse events. To do this, you have to pay attention to your internal dialogue and notice the knee-jerk responses that arise when something unwanted happens.

1. **Write down the adversity.**

2. **List the thoughts and beliefs that arise as a result
    of the adversity.**

3. **Record the consequences.** How did you feel? How
    did you behave?

4. **Review your patterns of belief and how they af-
    fect the consequences.** Are you a pessimist or an
    optimist? After reviewing the beliefs that arise in the
    face of adversity, pessimists may notice how the be-
    liefs that arise trigger negative emotional states or
    behaviors, whereas optimists may notice that their
    beliefs help them overcome adversity quickly.

5. **Dispute your pessimistic beliefs.** To do this, you
    have to learn how to argue with yourself. When ad-
    versity happens, notice any pessimistic beliefs that
    arise, then make a case to prove yourself wrong.
    If you automatically assume the worst, consider
    whether there are any other explanations for why
    adversity happened. Brainstorm other explanations
    for why your boss got upset or your boyfriend can-
    celed the date. Since you don't know for sure which
    ones are true, why not choose beliefs that help you
    feel more courageous and calm? Choose optimistic
    beliefs instead and notice whether they abort the
    downward spiral that pessimistic beliefs trigger.

Asking What's True

It's tempting to try to ditch *all* negative thoughts and beliefs,
but sometimes these thoughts are not just harming you—they're
helping you in some ways as well. This creates a paradox, and
leaning into paradox has the potential to loosen the grip of the
cognitive mind and make space for creative problem solving.

In Lisby's book *Extraordinary Knowing,* she tells the story of
her colleague Phyllis Cath, a highly regarded, very rational psy-
chiatrist. Lisby was telling Phyllis a story about a man who knew

something he shouldn't have known, in an extraordinary way that could only be attributed to a "sixth sense." Her friend's response was an experience of paradox: "On the one hand, listening to the story, I kept feeling, 'Of course!' But on the other, I'm completely amazed and find it unbelievable. How can I think both things at once? It makes no sense! In either mental framework, each is totally true . . . That story entered my mind in two ways at once and two ways that don't add up."

What happened to Phyllis Cath when she heard this story is that she entered the realm of paradox, where her thoughts registered in her mind as simultaneously both expectable and unbelievable. She was able to flip back and forth between two mutually incompatible points of view without reconciling them or having to decide which one was actually true. She neither rejected nor accepted either point of view. It's almost as if her mind had to open in order to hold both points of view at once. And when your mind opens in this way, it invites possibility in.

If you're not sure in what ways your beliefs are helping or limiting you, try examining them with a technique that my business partner, depth psychologist Anne Davin, Ph.D., uses with her clients: a practice of asking yourself what's true and what's not true about your beliefs.

COURAGE-CULTIVATING EXERCISE #17

What's True and What's Not True?

1. Examine the beliefs you're telling yourself in a situation. Perhaps your belief is "This will never pay the bills" or "I'm too old to do what I love." If you can, narrow your belief down to a single sentence. (If you have more than one belief, you can do this exercise many times.)

2. Examine what you wrote and ask yourself what's true about it. Call upon your Inner Pilot Light and put to use your powers of discernment to consider

---

which aspects are useful. In a separate list, write down what's true.

3. Examine what you wrote and ask yourself what's not true about what you wrote. Call upon your Inner Pilot Light and put to use your powers of discernment to consider which aspects are not useful. Write down what's not true.

4. Take a moment in silence with your eyes closed to allow your mind to hold both sides.

5. See if holding the paradox allows for any creative solutions to bubble up.

STEP 2: SUPPORT. *Seek out support from people around you—and offer your support to others.*

While cultivating courage is a self-guided process, it would be inaccurate to suggest that you can do it all alone. The journey from fear to courage is ultimately an intimate hero's journey, but every hero needs mentors, sidekicks, accountability partners, and cheerleaders. When you're trying to alchemize fear into growth, it's common to encounter well-meaning family, friends, and loved ones who are projecting their own fears onto you, rather than supporting your courageous choices. Not only does this make it hard to feel supported in those choices, it can also amplify your own fear. Fear begets fear, and when you're in the vulnerable beginning stages of this kind of transformation, you may need to work at creating a cocoon that nurtures and nourishes your courage instead.

In the same TED talk that I referenced in Chapter 2, Kelly McGonigal concluded that one healthy aspect of stress is that it makes you social by releasing oxytocin as part of the stress response. This "cuddle hormone" motivates you to seek support during scary, stressful times in your life—and this is a good thing. This is why Step 2 of the Six Steps to Cultivating Courage is all about social support. When life is scary, you need to be surrounded by people who care for you. But you'll also benefit from shifting your own focus to the service of others in trying times. The social connection works both ways. Receiving the love of others makes you brave, but so does caring for them.

Oxytocin doesn't just motivate you to seek out support when you're feeling scared and stressed. When you follow through, seeking out support instead of bottling up your emotions and keeping them to yourself, you release more oxytocin, and this hormone actually protects your cardiovascular system from the harmful effects of fear. Because it's a natural anti-inflammatory, it helps your blood vessels stay relaxed during stressful life events. Because your heart has oxytocin receptors, the hormone helps heart cells regenerate and heal from the damage of chronic stress responses. Oxytocin strengthens the heart, even in the face of fear, and you recover from scary emotions and stressful life events more quickly, not just on an emotional level, but physically.

One study tracked approximately 1,000 adults in the United States who ranged in age from 34 to 93. Study participants were asked how much stress they experienced in the last year. They were also asked how much time they spent helping out friends, neighbors, and people in their community. Then researchers used public records over the next five years to find out who among them died during that time.

What they found is that for every stressful life experience, such as a death in the family or a financial crisis, the risk of dying increased by 30 percent. But this scary number didn't apply to all the study participants. People who spent time caring for others demonstrated no stress-related increase in dying. Caring for others—and being cared for—created resilience.

When you change your beliefs—Step 1 in the process of cultivating courage—and are able to view loss and uncertainty in new ways, so that they become opportunities for growth and connection, you become resilient, both emotionally and physically. And when you use these experiences as an opportunity to seek support and serve others, you amplify this resilience. In effect, you're creating the biology of courage. This is why Step 2 is all about seeking out the right social support, as well as offering social support to others from the heart. Let's start by considering how you'll find the right social support; then we'll discuss how you might give it to others as a way to ramp up your courage.

What Does "Everybody" Think?

Part of what may hold you back from courageous action is your fear of what "Everybody" will think if you take risks that may look "crazy" to other people. Keep in mind that what you consider brave, everyone else may indeed consider crazy—and that's often how you know you're on the right track. In any case, who is this Everybody you're so worried about? In *Finding Your Own North Star,* Martha Beck teaches that most people's Everybody is composed of just a few key people. Because we are social creatures who feel safe in tribes, we will do whatever we can to fit into the clan. But it's hard to hold the tastes and opinions of more than five or six individuals in your mind at once, so instead of choosing to make up our own minds, the resourceful part of you that yearns for approval from the tribe creates a kind of shorthand. It selects the attitudes and opinions of a few key players, whom psychologists term "the generalized other," imprints these judgments on your brain, and extrapolates this small smattering of Everybody to represent the whole entire planet of human beings who are surely sitting there just waiting to make you wrong.

Instead of worrying about what Everybody will think if we do something brave, Martha invites us to create a new Everybody by building an inner circle of trustworthy advisors, people whose opinions we know we can trust.

Courage-Cultivating Exercise #18

Create Your New "Everybody"

1. **Name your current Everybody.** List the names of all the people whose judgment or approval you're thinking of when you worry about what Everybody will think.

2. **Notice whether these people model qualities you wish to emulate.** Are they kind? Filled with integrity? Compassionate? Brave? Don't judge these people, but do ask yourself whether you really value their opinions.

3. **Choose your ideal Everybody.** Perhaps some of the people in your current Everybody are there because you value and respect their counsel. If so, keep them! But if these people limit you more than they facilitate your growth, you can choose a brand-new Everybody. The good news is that you don't even have to know these people personally. For that matter, they don't even have to be alive. You can call upon the wisdom of others, living or dead, whether you know them in the flesh or not. These may be real people who love and support you and have your best interests at heart. They may be authors who have written inspiring books, spiritual teachers living or dead, or even angels or deities. Choose six people who unconditionally encourage you and help you feel more brave.

4. **Consult your new Everybody regularly.** Ask for advice in meditation, in writing, in prayer, or in person whenever you need genuinely helpful guidance.

Adapted from the Find Your Calling teleclass I teach with Martha Beck and Amy Ahlers, based on Martha's book *Finding Your Own North Star.*

Finding Aligned Mentors

In the process of cultivating courage, finding the right mentor who is at least a few steps ahead of you on your journey of transformation can change everything. Some of these mentors may be people you include in your Everybody. The key is to find mentors you can trust to buoy the part of you that yearns to make decisions from courage and trust, rather than fear.

Finding the right mentors can be tricky. You may not find one mentor who can hold your hand through every step of your personal journey, but if you're willing to let go and trust, you may find that the perfect mentor appears right on your doorstep or in your e-mail inbox at the perfect time. And if you move beyond one mentor, the next may be right there, holding out a hand to guide you.

You may find an aligned mentor:

- At a place of worship
- Through an elder in your life
- By asking a trusted friend to refer you to a spiritual teacher
- Through the books, blogs, teleclasses, lectures, or videos of teachers you don't necessarily know personally
- By following your intuitive guidance and hiring someone who works one-on-one with clients as a transpersonal psychologist, spiritual counselor, therapist, or coach
- By asking a yoga, meditation, or spiritual teacher you trust
- By participating in a spiritual community and meeting someone a few steps ahead of you on his or her own journey who volunteers to help you
- As your sponsor in a 12-step program

- If you're lucky, you may find the kinds of relationships that spiritual teacher Craig Hamilton calls "evolutionary relationships," which may be lovers, friends, family members, or colleagues who agree to be in relationship with you in a potentially uncomfortable, challenging, but loving way that is based on the shared desire to move beyond your false fears and align with your highest self.

COURAGE-CULTIVATING EXERCISE #19

How to Find an Aligned Mentor

1. **Ask that the right mentor appear.** They say that when the student is ready, the teacher appears. When the teacher is ready, the student appears. Such unions may happen spontaneously and feel divinely guided, but you can also pray for guidance. Get clear on your intention to find a mentor, pray for guidance, let go of your attachment to outcomes, then pay attention to the guidance that appears.

2. **State your intention to others.** Let people you trust know you're seeking the right mentor for your journey. Ask for referrals. If you know someone on a spiritual path who has benefited from the support of a spiritual mentor, find out whether that person would be willing to mentor you as well. You might even find the right person by announcing your desire on social media or sending out an e-mail to those you trust. Allowing your desire to be known publicly can facilitate the process.

3. **Be willing to be surprised.** Your mentor might be an established spiritual teacher or a professional counselor. She could be a well-known author or an ordained minister. He might lead transformational workshops or host spiritual gatherings. But keep your mind and heart open because the right mentor might not be who you expect. Your mentor might be younger than you. She might be an elderly woman in a nursing home. He could be a homeless man who spouts wisdom when you visit him on his park bench. She could be your boss or your house-

keeper. Don't limit your mentorship opportunities with narrow expectations.

4. **Trust your instincts and your body.** Look for that "plunk of truth" in your gut when you meet the right person. Pay attention to the people whose words give you goose bumps, because *your body knows they speak truth.*

5. **Be bold.** If you meet someone who lights up your soul, don't hesitate to ask if he or she would be willing to offer you guidance. If someone says no, don't take it personally. Trust that whatever the answer is, it's aligned with your highest good, and know that the right mentor will appear in divine timing.

Don't forget that you can always mentor yourself. Within you lies the wise, loving, discerning mentorship of your Inner Pilot Light. Not sure what to do next? Ask your Inner Pilot Light. Once you learn to access this unfailing part of you, you will realize that you never need to be separated from your inner guidance. We'll talk more about how to receive and interpret this essential guidance in Step 3.

Finding Your Soul Community

Especially if you perceive that your old Everybody will judge you if you align with your truth, it's critical to the success of your journey to surround yourself with a community of people dedicated to living the kind of courageous life you are committed to living. Your soul community can lift you up, give you accountability, increase your commitment to living courageously, and mirror back to you where you're on track and where your growth edges are.

OPPORTUNITIES FOR SOUL COMMUNITY

- Communities of worship, like a church, a temple, a mosque, or a Zen center

- Classes based on a shared spiritual interest, such as meditation, developing your intuition, or embracing the Divine Feminine or Divine Masculine

- Spiritually based conferences, such as Hay House's I Can Do It! conferences, Wisdom 2.0, Health & Harmony Festival, and Wild Goose Festival

- Yoga classes

- Ecstatic dance communities

- Volunteer organizations

- Women's and men's groups

- Gatherings at retreat centers like Esalen Institute, Kripalu, and Omega Institute

- Meditation circles

- Spiritual, religious, or metaphysical bookstores

- 12-step programs

- School groups, such as college clubs or a group of like-minded parents who gather from your child's school

- Certification programs, such as the Whole Health Medicine Institute program I lead, or Martha Beck's life coaching program

- Spiritually based virtual programs, such as my Medicine for the Soul, Find Your Calling, and Visionary Ignition Switch programs, Craig Hamilton's Integral Enlightenment, or Tosha Silver's Offerings class

- Facebook groups

- Online forums

- Blog communities

- Musical groups, such as drum circles, kirtan chanting groups, and choirs

- Spiritually minded professional groups, such as the Finding Meaning in Medicine groups Rachel Naomi Remen helps organize for physicians

- Study groups based on sacred texts, such as Bible study or *A Course in Miracles* study groups

- Book clubs dedicated to reading spiritually based books

- Inspirational exercise groups, such as SoulCycle

- Consult the tips from Anne Davin, Ph.D., for creating your own soul community in Appendix C: 7 Steps for Creating Your Tribe

Serve Others

While finding the right support is essential to cultivating courage, focusing exclusively on the self in a fear-based way can limit your capacity to be brave. It's essential to meet your own needs first in a healthy way so your service to others comes from a pure place, stemming from your sense of connection with all beings rather than from some sort of codependent "savior complex." Once you are giving to others from this pure place of genuine service, your nervous system will relax, your fear will subside, and your courage will grow.

Andy Mackie demonstrated this well. Faced with his own looming death after nine heart surgeries that failed to cure him, Andy was on 15 medications as his doctors tried to save his life. But the side effects of the drugs made him miserable. He finally made the courageous decision to stop all his medications and spend his remaining days doing something he had always wanted to do instead. Even though his doctors insisted he would die within a year, Andy decided to use the money he would have spent on his heart medicines to purchase 300 harmonicas and give them away to children, complete with lessons from Andy. When he was still alive a month later, he bought a few hundred more. Thirteen years and 20,000 harmonicas later, Andy Mackie finally passed away in 2012. The Andy Mackie Music Foundation still carries on his vision.

Sometimes what makes us most brave requires us to do something scary not for ourselves, but on behalf of others. Andy Mackie's brave service allowed him to overcome his fear of dying enough to stop the medications that were causing him to suffer. By focusing on the children he would serve instead of his own fear of death, he helped others, and as he did so, his own health improved. Since fear tends to inspire us to reach out in order to comfort ourselves, we might as well utilize this natural social inclination to channel our fear into this kind of service. In this way, fear can actually motivate us to make the world a better place.

Chris Guillebeau was inspired to a service-oriented life after the fear-inducing events of September 11 fueled him to move to Africa in order to help others on a hospital ship. Ten years later, in 2011, he kicked off the first World Domination Summit, a conference intended to help visionaries amplify their service in the world. He hosted the conference at a personal loss of about $30,000. Chris didn't mind that he lost money on the event. It was his own act of service. The following year, a private donor who heard that Chris lost money on the first conference offered to help fund the next one. A savvy businessman, Chris had already figured out how to not only break even the next year, but also turn a profit. With the combined profits and the large anonymous donation, Chris could have paid himself back for 2011's losses and put some away for future conferences. Instead, Chris chose to do something remarkable.

When he did the math, it turned out that the $100,000 donation, divided by the number of attendees at the conference (1,000), came out to exactly $100 per person. Chris, who had just written a book called *The $100 Startup,* had an idea. At the end of the conference, which I attended, we were each handed an envelope. In it was a crisp $100 bill. Under the words *The $100 Investment,* a note on the envelope read, *We'd love to see how you can put these funds to good use. Start a project, surprise someone, or do something entirely different—it's up to you.*

I spent the next few days marinating on how I would utilize my $100 investment. I decided to write a blog post inviting my readers to share with me *their* ideas about how they would use $100 to make the world a better place. I would pick the most inspiring idea and donate my $100 to that reader. Hundreds of readers shared their ideas about what they would do with $100 to change the world. Some were so inspired by other readers' ideas that they offered to donate their $100 to fund those. The whole thing exploded. Together, the readers wound up investing thousands of dollars in world-changing ideas, while I watched the whole thing unfold, moved to tears by the generosity of strangers who were so committed to service.

So I'll leave you with the next Courage-Cultivating Exercise as a challenge of your own courage. Do you have $100 you could invest in something bigger than yourself?

Courage-Cultivating Exercise #20

The $100 Investment

1. If someone gave you $100 and charged you to go and make the world a better place, what would you do with it?

2. Can you spare $100 of your own money to put your plan into action? Are you brave enough to do so?

3. If you don't have $100 to spare, can you brainstorm ways to raise $100? Are there others who might be willing to fund you?

4. Can you challenge someone else to change the world with $100? Would they be willing to meet the challenge with you? Imagine if every person who could afford it invested $100 in making the world a better place . . .

STEP 3: INTUITION. *Learn to trust your intuition in order to discern true fear from false fear.*

Once you can differentiate between true fear and false fear, you can trust that your instincts will alert you to the true fears that need immediate action, so you can question and examine your false fears and let them fuel your growth without letting them guide your decisions. The more you can do this, the more you can cultivate courage. As long as the amygdala is on high alert, triggering stress responses an average of 50 times per day, making courageous choices can be challenging. When the nervous system calms down, it's easier to access your brave.

In order to distinguish between true fear and false fear, it's essential to tap into and trust your Inner Pilot Light, which speaks in the voice of your intuition and sends you valuable guidance signals via your body. Although we are wired to pay attention to intuition, our culture does not value it. Often, we scoff at it, dismiss it, and relegate it to the realm of those psychics I mentioned earlier, with crystal balls and muumuus. And many of us aren't living truly embodied lives; we only live in the vicinities of our bodies. We've become so caught up in our heads and dissociated from the signals our bodies send that we ignore this inner compass.

Discerning True Fear from False Fear

As we saw in Chapter 3, the easiest way to discern whether fear is true or false is to determine whether someone is in danger in present time. Is there a wild animal chasing you? Is someone about to drown at the beach? Is your child at risk of injury or death? Has it been days since you or a loved one have had enough food? Might you die in the next few minutes? These would all be obvious true fears. True fear triggers ACTION. It says, "Do something—now!" In these situations, your body activates appropriate stress responses that help protect you and those around you. You won't have to think about whether or not to act—you just will. If you watch your baby fall into a swimming pool, or you see someone get shot, or your mother screams out in terror from the back room, you will do something about it without having to think.

But true fear isn't always this cut-and-dried. Sometimes it shows up in more subtle—and potentially confusing—ways. True fear can also show up as an intuitive knowing that says, *I'm not letting my child spend the night at that person's house.* It can show up as a dream, an inner voice, or a gut feeling that something bad is about to happen. These examples of intuitive knowing don't necessarily reflect an immediate threat in present time, but the fear they carry may indeed be true fear. And they may lead you to alter your behavior in ways that protect against real danger. You might walk into a room with a stranger, and even though the stranger seems perfectly friendly, you may feel the urge to get the hell outta Dodge. Or you might have a dream about getting in a car accident that leads you to take extra precautions the next time you get in a car. Larry Burk, M.D., a radiologist, is collecting stories of patients whose breast cancer was diagnosed and treated because they heeded the messages of warning dreams. Countless stories of parents' intuition helping to protect their children suggest that this kind of true fear may be particularly strong with regard to those we love most.

The root of the word *intuition* is *tuere,* which means "to guard, to protect." Intuition functions not just to protect us, but to protect others. In my work as a physician, my intuition has protected my patients countless times. You'll hear the same thing from any cop or soldier. This is why paying attention to true fear is so important.

But how do you know which fears to pay attention to and which ones to ignore? This is where Gavin de Becker's wisdom comes in handy. De Becker, author of *The Gift of Fear,* is a three-time presidential appointee who runs a firm that consults with the government, law enforcement agencies, and prominent media figures, teaching about how to accurately assess threats of violence.

In de Becker's experience, victims of violent crimes almost always say they felt afraid just before a criminal harmed them, yet they ignored these feelings because the fear seemed irrational. From what their cognitive minds could determine, the fear had no basis. Before the violence began, the criminal seemed polite, helpful, and safe. Yet the victims were being alerted by a highly sensitive and accurate internal warning system.

As de Becker instructs, when our lives are in danger, gut (intuition) trumps head (cognition) every time. He explains, "We think conscious thought is somehow better, when in fact, intuition is soaring flight compared to the plodding of logic. Nature's greatest accomplishment, the human brain, is never more efficient and invested than when its host is at risk. Then, intuition is catapulted to another level entirely, a height at which it can accurately be called graceful, even miraculous. Intuition is the journey from A to Z without stopping at any other letter along the way. It is knowing without knowing why . . . Intuition is always learning, and though it may occasionally send a signal that turns out to be less than urgent, everything it communicates to you is meaningful. Unlike worry, it will not waste your time. Intuition might send any of several messengers to get your attention, and because they differ according to urgency, it is good to know the ranking."

De Becker explains that intuition speaks to us in a sort of hierarchy of urgency, with fear at the top of the urgency pyramid, followed by—in this order—apprehension, suspicion, hesitation, doubt, gut feelings, hunches, and curiosity. You might also experience nagging feelings, persistent thoughts, physical sensations, wonder, anxiety, or even a flash of dark humor. De Becker says, "By thinking about these signals with an open mind when they occur, you will learn how you communicate with yourself."

How Intuition Feels

Discerning between true and false fear requires learning to identify how intuition shows up for you. As part of my research for this book, I interviewed many people who had experienced intuitive hunches that protected them or someone else, including the examples I shared in Chapter 6. When I asked people how they knew to pay attention to the hunches and how they differentiated these hunches from paranoid thoughts, most said that they didn't actually feel scared when the hunch came in. Even though a premonition might have presented a scary image to the mind, their reaction was often not a feeling of panic, but one of profound calm. In fact, those who have really developed their intuition report that this inner stillness is often what helps them discern whether an intuitive feeling is real. Others find that the body helps with discernment. Fear often shows up as a gripping feeling in the solar plexus, whereas intuition often comes with a feeling of inner spaciousness, even relaxation. How does your intuition speak to you through your body?

COURAGE-CULTIVATING EXERCISE #21

Use Body Awareness to Discern True Fear from False Fear

1. **Consider a fearful thought that you're having trouble defining as true or false fear.** Maybe your fear feels like an instinct meant to protect you, but you're not convinced it's not just anxiety or paranoia.

2. **Let your body really feel the fearful thought.** Don't just think it in your mind. Sense it in your body. Let it infuse you.

---

3. **Notice your body's reaction to the fearful thought.** Do you feel panicky or calm? Is your heart racing or steady? Is your breathing rapid or slow? Do you feel tight or relaxed in your solar plexus? Do you feel pain anywhere, or does your body feel open? Ask your body whether it has any messages for you. Pay particular attention to how your body feels.

4. **Bring your body into relaxation response and come into present time.** You can employ any technique that works for you, such as meditation, EFT, yoga, or deep breathing.

5. **From this place of deep physical relaxation and presence, try to sense the quality of the fearful thought.** Can you feel calm, relaxed, present, and still engaged with the thought? Are you still worried, anxious, or afraid when you think this thought? Or does the thought lose its power when your body is relaxed and your mind is resting in the present moment? If the fearful thought loses its edge when you're calm and present, it's probably a false fear that's safe to ignore. If the thought still feels potent and true, even when you're calm, it's more likely to be your intuition communicating a message of protection that's worth noting.

Turning Up the Volume

Some people feel more naturally tapped into their intuition than others, but everyone has the capacity to be intuitive. Often, traumatic experiences in childhood, such as child abuse and sexual molestation, will heighten a child's intuition as a way of protecting the child from more danger. These children may grow up to be naturally intuitive in a way that children who grow up feeling safe don't need. Some children are *born* highly intuitive and are allowed to develop their intuition without others making it "wrong." Others may have their intuition questioned; parents may tell them they're "silly" or "making things up" if they share evidence of strong intuitive skills. These children, feeling unsafe, may "go cognitive" and push intuition underground, making it more difficult to access.

The good news is that, like courage and optimism, intuition can be cultivated. Try some of the following tips to turn up the volume on that inner voice.

How to Strengthen Your Intuition

- **Meditate.** Messages from your intuition tend to be quiet, so spending time in silence will help you hear and interpret these messages.

- **Develop your sensory awareness.** Start noticing all that you can with your five conventional senses. Doing so can raise your sensitivity to your sixth sense.

- **Pay attention to your dreams.** When the cognitive mind is busy, it can override the intuitive right brain and the subconscious mind, the wellspring of intuition. But when you're sleeping, your cognitive mind rests and opens space for the subconscious mind to signal you in dreams.

- **Get creative.** Engaging in creative activities, such as drawing, scrapbooking, or free-flow journaling, quiets the cognitive mind and allows your intuition to speak up.

- **Consult oracle cards.** Learn to use a Tarot deck or try a deck of oracle cards, such as Doreen Virtue's Goddess Guidance Oracle Cards.

- **Test your hunches.** Got a feeling which horse will win at the track? Getting a sense that it will rain tomorrow even though the weather forecast says it won't? Do you just *know* your best friend's new guy is bad news? If you have feelings about what might happen in the future, write down your hunches, then check them later. See how often you were right.

- **Consult your body compass.** Your intuition speaks to you through your body, and the more you cultivate somatic awareness, the more sensitive you become. If you get an uncomfortable physical feeling when you're trying to make a decision, pay attention. Do you feel light or heavy? Got a sick feeling in your gut? Saddled with a headache or diarrhea? It could just be the result of stress responses activated by false fear, but it could also be your intuition ringing loud and clear.

- **Escape from your daily routine.** Get away. Slow down. Go on a retreat, take a sabbatical, or just spend a day in new surroundings with nothing planned. When you're overly busy, it's hard to be sensitive to the quiet voices of intuition. Try clearing your schedule and see if your intuition pipes up.

- **Spend time in nature.** Being in the natural world, away from technology and the cognitive mind's other temptations, can open up the kind of intuition we needed when we as a species lived outdoors and relied upon it to keep us safe from the elements, predators, and other true fear dangers.

- **Learn from the past.** Recall a negative experience from your past, ideally something fairly recent. Before this thing happened, think back to whether you got any feelings that urged you to steer clear. Maybe you got a gut feeling something wasn't right. Maybe you had a foreshadowing dream or a vision. If so, did you pay attention to that feeling, dream, or vision, or did you talk yourself out of it? Try to remember exactly how you felt. Recall as many details as possible. The more you can get in touch with the part of you that tried to warn you, the more you'll trust it next time.

- **Feel, don't think.** The mind thinks, always chattering away, arguing with itself like a crazy person. Intuition, on the other hand, feels. If you're not sure whether you're listening to your fearful mind or your trustworthy intuition, see if you can differentiate whether you're thinking or feeling.

- **Engage in repetitive movement.** Run. Dance. Chop carrots. Play the piano. Paint. These physical actions can calm the cognitive mind and open up your intuition.

- **Align with your values.** Your mind may steer you away from your integrity, but your intuition never will. Become comfortable with how you feel when you're betraying your values, and you'll learn what intuition doesn't feel like. Learn what it feels like to behave in alignment with your values, and you'll start to sense your intuition more clearly.

- **Practice sensing into people before you know them.** See what kind of information you can glean from observing people and feeling their energetic signature before you talk to them or learn anything about them from other people. The more you pay attention, the more you'll realize you already know things you couldn't possibly know with the cognitive mind.

- **Read books about how to develop your intuition.** Try Sonia Choquette's *Trust Your Vibes,* Shakti Gawain's *Developing Intuition,* or Caroline Myss's *Sacred Contracts.*

- **Train your intuition.** You can study intuition in formal classroom settings, as well as online programs. Try the Academy of Intuition Medicine, the Foundation for Spiritual Development, or Jenai Lane's Spirit Coach training program.

- **Release your resistance.** Don't call yourself crazy when you get an intuitive hunch. Often, the cognitive mind argues with intuition rather than trusting it. By doing this, you may rationalize yourself out of intuitive knowing that could save your life.

Getting to Know Your Inner Pilot Light

You already know that the part of you I call the Inner Pilot Light—your guide on this whole courage-cultivating journey—is speaking from your intuition. So a powerful way to discern true fear from false fear is to work at cultivating your relationship with this part of you. If you have trouble communicating with your Inner Pilot Light, try the following practices to get better acquainted.

- **Get quiet.** It's almost impossible to hear the voice of your Inner Pilot Light when your environment is noisy and your mind is busy. In meditation, ask your Inner Pilot Light to share with you any wisdom it might have for you today.

- **Read the Daily Flame.** These daily messages are love letters from your Inner Pilot Light to your Small Self. Sign up at InnerPilotLight.com. Or write your own!

- **Let your Inner Pilot Light write a letter to your wounded child self.** Think of the hardest time from your childhood, a time when you felt very hurt, lonely, scared, angry, or disappointed. Let your Inner Pilot Light offer love and guidance to this wounded part of you.

- **Go on a hike with your Inner Pilot Light.** Set the intention from the beginning that you are open to receiving guidance. Then pay attention. Notice. Listen.

- **Invite your Inner Pilot Light to choose your dreams.** Let it speak to you in dream time and help you interpret your dreams when you wake up.

- **Draw your Inner Pilot Light.** What does this part of you look like? Engage your most creative self. Use pencil, colored markers, crayons, paints, or whatever lights you up.

- **Let your Inner Pilot Light make you a vision board.** Cut out words and images from magazines and paste them on a sheet of paper. Don't question what your Inner Pilot Light picks.

- **Invite your Inner Pilot Light to choose a mantra or affirmation for you.** Pick something like "I'm on the right path, even if I don't know where I'm going," or "It's safe to let go of false fear," or "I am enough."

- **Make an Inner Pilot Light reading list.** What books light up this part of you?

- **Make an Inner Pilot Light friend list.** Who are the people that activate this part of you?

- **Make an Inner Pilot Light place list.** What are the places that fan the flames of your Inner Pilot Light?

- **Make an Inner Pilot Light playlist.** What music makes your Inner Pilot Light come alive?

- **Choose your Inner Pilot Light wardrobe.** If your Inner Pilot Light could dress you, how would this part of you advise you to dress? What's your Inner Pilot Light's favorite color? Pick at least one outfit that makes you feel illuminated.

- **Meet your Inner Pilot Light in a guided meditation.** For a guided meditation of me leading you through the process of meeting your inner wise mentor, download the free Prescription for Courage Kit at TheFearCureBook.com.

You can also ask your Inner Pilot Light to have a heart-to-heart conversation with your Small Self. I often engage in this kind of dialogue. By recognizing that the fear is just the part of me that's trying to protect me, I can compassionately argue with it, and as I do, it loses some of its power. I can also examine it for areas of growth that might need my attention. For example, if I'm afraid to initiate a vulnerable conversation with someone I care about, the dialogue might go something like this.

Small Self: *You can't say that. He'll think you're "too much" and run screaming in the other direction like all the other guys have.*

Inner Pilot Light: *Well, that's one possible outcome, and if that happens, then that's useful research about the strength of this relationship. Another possible outcome is that if you express honest feelings, he'll understand your feelings better and choose to meet you more consciously.*

Small Self: *Yeah, right. On some other planet, maybe. But on this one, you know how guys respond when you get vulnerable. They see you as weak and needy, and then they freak out and leave, and you're left with a broken heart. You should have learned by now that you should just keep these thoughts to yourself.*

Inner Pilot Light: *Well, maybe you've been weak and needy. You have a tendency to get that way when you're in charge. But I'm in charge, and he has always held our vulnerability gently. We've earned this person's trust, and he's earned ours. Think back to all the times we've shared something vulnerable with him and he's held that vulnerability gently, without running away. Do you really think he's going to reject us when we're speaking our truth? Even if that has happened in the past, it doesn't mean it's going to happen now. Plus, remember our values. Speaking our truth with those who have earned our trust is a core value of ours. Let's not sacrifice our values just because you're afraid of getting hurt. Let me tell him how you feel. Worst-case scenario, he rejects us, and if that's the case, you'll always have me. I will never abandon you. Best-case scenario, we build even more trust and intimacy because he has demonstrated that he can hold our vulnerability with care. Even if you wind up hurt, remember that we value being brave, and sharing how you feel is the courageous thing to do.*

Another way to dialogue directly with your fear and call forth the voice of your Inner Pilot Light is to write letters between the two. Like the Small Self conversation, this can give you the distance you need to realize that fear is only one voice inside of you. This can be very helpful as a way to let fear fuel your growth and deliver any messages about what's in need of healing. Here's an example of how that might look.

> *Dear Liz,*
>
> *Don't you remember what happened when we let others take control of our life? We weren't safe. Mom was always on the verge of walking out. Dad was always drinking. You were always getting beaten. We wound up first living with Grandma, then bouncing around foster homes. Don't you see that I'm only trying to protect you? If you don't listen to me, all hell will break loose. I care about you. I just want you to stay safe. Please listen to me. You can trust me to take care of you when you can't trust anyone else. I'm always here for you. You need me.*
>
> *Loving and protecting you,*
>
> *Fear*

And here's how the Inner Pilot Light might respond.

> *Dear Fear,*
>
> *I hear you, darling. Thank you for taking care of us all those years ago. We might not have survived if you hadn't protected us. You saved us then. But things are different now. I'm here, all grown up. I can take care of you. You don't have to be afraid anymore. You're safe. I'm on it. Things will not fall apart if you trust me. In fact, if you're able to let me take over, everything you think you want will suddenly be available to us. We'll be able to love bigger, dream bigger, risk bigger, and make a difference in the world. But I can't do this unless you're on board with me. I won't leave you. I want you with me, but I need you to let go and trust me. You can let go now. You are safe. Liz is safe. We are safe. All is well.*
>
> *Gratefully,*
>
> *Your Inner Pilot Light*

The more we try to resist Fear, the louder and scarier Fear can become. But when we befriend Fear instead, it can calm down. Ask Fear why it's here. Let it make a case for how it's trying to help you. Listen to where Fear is coming from. Honor the part of you that has been hurt in the past and is just trying to protect you.

Don't judge Fear. Don't get angry at Fear. Don't try to silence Fear. It doesn't work. Instead, invite your Inner Pilot Light to be compassionate with Fear. Be loving. Be patient. Let Fear know you're not trying to get rid of it; you just don't want it in the driver's seat anymore. Let Fear cure you, if you're brave enough.

The next exercise allows you to dialogue back and forth between Fear and your Inner Pilot Light yourself.

COURAGE-CULTIVATING EXERCISE #22

Write a Letter from Your Inner Pilot Light

1. **Close your eyes, focus on your breath, and let your mind quiet down.**

2. **Invite Fear to write you a letter.** Start with *Dear YOU,* and end with *Love, Fear.* Don't censor this. Let Fear get as scary, whiny, nasty, childish, and weak as it can.

3. **Now sense the presence of your Inner Pilot Light.** Feel this wise, loving mentor within. Let it nurture you. Be held by your highest self.

4. **Ask your Inner Pilot Light to respond to Fear.** Start with *Dear Fear,* and end with *Love, Your Inner Pilot Light.* If you can align with this part of yourself, you can completely trust the guidance you receive. But don't get tricked! Your fearful Small Self can try to hijack any inner voice you come to trust. The Small Self LOVES to masquerade as the voice of wisdom and hide behind the mask of "protector." Be very clear with your intentions. Ask that only your Inner Pilot Light be allowed to write. If the voice is self-critical, judging, frightened, doubtful, bossy, suspicious, or ruminating on negative thoughts, this is not your Inner Pilot Light. The voice of your Inner Pilot Light may not always tell you what you want to hear, but it will have the ring of truth to it. Most notably, it will always feel loving and compassionate, even if it's telling you to steer clear of something or someone potentially dangerous.

> 5. **If you feel inspired to do so, let Fear write back again.** See if Fear has any more messages for you that will point you to your growth edges. Then, if you want to, allow your Inner Pilot Light to respond in writing to Fear. Let the dialogue go on as long as you need it to in order to gain clarity about what Fear is trying to teach you.

STEP 4: DIAGNOSE. *Identify what lies at the root of your false fear.*

The crux of The Fear Cure lies in letting fear illuminate the obstacles between you and inner peace. What still needs to be healed within you? What predisposes you to fearful thoughts? What influences from your childhood trigger false fears that may still be operating you? How might your unconscious be driving you to be unnecessarily afraid? What people amplify your false fear? Your answers to these questions can help you make your "Fear Diagnosis." Diagnosing the root causes of your fear raises your awareness so fear can no longer hide out in the shadows of your consciousness and run your life without your permission. By gently and compassionately outing the roots of your fears, you bring them into the light, where they automatically begin to dissipate in the brightness of your awareness.

For most of us, if we dig deep enough down to those roots, we find one or more (or all) of the Four Fearful Assumptions:

1. Uncertainty is unsafe.
2. I can't handle losing what I cherish.
3. It's a dangerous world.
4. I am all alone.

Being able to recognize that you're unnecessarily afraid because you're making one or more of these assumptions can help you abort the false fear downward spiral. Practicing the exercises in Part Two of this book so you can start operating from the Four Courage-Cultivating Truths instead of the Four Fearful Assumptions will help you operate from a braver worldview. Changing your worldview may change everything, and you may find your day-to-day fears loosening their grip. Or you may still find yourself struggling with them. Understanding what predisposes you to these fears can help you heal from the root of what lies beneath them. Awareness of your Fear Diagnosis can also assist you when it comes time to write your Prescription for Courage.

TEN COMMON FALSE FEAR ROOTS

1. Limiting beliefs arising from childhood, such as the belief that there's never enough to go around

2. Generational fears, which tend to get passed down from our parents and theirs before them

3. Memories of past dangers we have faced

4. Projections of the fearful imagination into the future

5. Instinctual fears, such as a fear of snakes or heights—basic survival fears that all humans have to some degree

6. Inadequate social support or mentorship

7. Pessimistic explanatory style

8. Fear-inducing religious upbringing

9. Exposure and sensitivity to the excessively fear-inducing media

10. Loss of spiritual connection

You may not realize it, but as we discussed in Chapter 3, you probably inherited most of your false fears. They were probably downloaded into your subconscious mind in your very early years. Your parents and others who influenced you at that age programmed you to be afraid. But it's not fair to blame them. Most of them are simply passing along these generational fears the way you might pass on a virus. They inherited these fears from their parents, and then you inherited yours from them. Because most of us aren't even aware of the fears that are driving our lives, we pass them on unconsciously to our own children. If you do the heavy lifting to heal your own false fears, you not only free yourself; you break the chain, disrupt the pattern of generational fears, spare your children, and heal future generations.

When you're carrying generational fear, it's easy to slip into the role of the victim. Such a feeling is understandable! The fear doesn't even belong to you; you inherited it from someone else. But it's important to realize you are not a victim. You are a survivor. When you see yourself that way, the generational fears you've carried don't cripple you. They strengthen you.

COURAGE-CULTIVATING EXERCISE #23

Break the Chain of Generational Fear

1. Pick a date when you feel ready, and tell yourself that for the next seven days after that, you are not allowed to be afraid.

2. If fear comes up (it will), ask yourself where that fear comes from. Are you mirroring your mother's fear? Are you rebelling against your father's fear? Is the fear really yours?

3. Regardless of where the fear comes from, set it aside for one week. Remind yourself that you're not allowed to be afraid and go to the next emotion. Maybe you're afraid to make changes in your marriage, but if you're not allowed to be afraid, what emotion do you feel next? Do you feel guilt?

Shame? Sadness? Frustration? Helplessness? If you're afraid about making changes at work, what would you feel if you weren't allowed to be afraid? What other emotions underlie your fears?

4. At the end of a week, make a note in your journal about how this experience went for you. Did you realize anything about the source of the fears you're carrying?

Your Operating Principles

Another way to pin down your Fear Diagnosis is to recognize how fear can hold you hostage without you even realizing it. To help students in the Medicine for the Soul teleclass identify how fear was driving their decisions, Rachel Naomi Remen and I invited them to consider what we called the "Small Self Operating Principles." Some examples of common Small Self Operating Principles include:

- Never, ever venture into the unknown.

- Don't share your truth.

- Do what you're told and you'll be loved.

- Prioritize what makes money, even if it makes you unhappy.

- Self-sacrifice is good. Self-care is selfish.

- Make no mistakes ever.

- Never disappoint anyone.

- Tell people what they want to hear.

- Avoid conflict at all costs.

- Perfect is the only thing that's good enough.

- Be in control at all times.

Every one of these Small Self Operating Principles—most of which stem from generational fears—is a barrier to living a courageous life. They get in the way of living your truth and following the guidance of your Inner Pilot Light—and when you're not doing that, things don't go well. Consider the times you've ignored your Inner Pilot Light. Chances are good that you made the choices that you did because you thought you were doing "the right thing"; chances are you were motivated by fear of disappointing people, fear of financial difficulty, fear of rejection, or other fears that led you to betray what was really true for you.

Maybe the wedding invites were already sent, so you figured you should go through with the wedding. Maybe you spent so many years training for the job you knew you wanted to leave—or the money or the security was so alluring—that you talked yourself out of your truth. Maybe you thought you were being a "good person" by taking care of the elderly relative who treated you like dirt. Maybe you worked yourself to death to pay for the quality of life you thought your family needed, when your Inner Pilot Light was telling you to simplify and downsize. Maybe you told yourself their quality of life was more important than yours.

Maybe your Inner Pilot Light doesn't want to go to church anymore, but your Small Self says you should. Maybe your Inner Pilot Light doesn't want to hang out with the friend you've known for 20 years, but your Small Self feels obligated by your history. Maybe your Inner Pilot Light doesn't like the missionary position and wants to get down and dirty, but your Small Self says it's not safe to let on that you fantasize the way you do. Maybe your Inner Pilot Light wants to dance under the moonlight, but your Small Self pushes you to the gym to lift weights at dawn instead. Your Inner Pilot Light wants to eat consciously raised meat, but your Small Self says you should be vegan. Your Inner Pilot Light is desperate for sleep, but your Small Self tells you you'll never get what you want if you sleep eight hours a night. Your Inner Pilot Light wants you to abide by its guidance, but your Small Self tells you this guidance can't be trusted. Your Small Self wants you to obey its Operating Principles *at all costs*. It's terrified of what would happen if you ever changed the rules. But aren't you curious? What if there was another way to live?

COURAGE-CULTIVATING EXERCISE #24

Your Operating Principles

- **List your Small Self Operating Principles.** What limiting rules are you living by? If you can't think of anything, consider what you believe is right and wrong. Reflect back to the rules your parents taught you. What rules do you teach your children? What did you learn in the church or temple or mosque about how to live? What do you believe you have to do to get love? Success? Health? Money? Security? Write down any beliefs or rules that come up.

- **List your Inner Pilot Light's Operating Principles.** Now consider who you are at your deepest core. What really matters to you? What do you yearn for? What do you really believe about what's right or wrong? What are your core values? What principles are aligned with your soul's integrity?

- **Compare the two lists.** You're bound to see discrepancies! Which list drives your life? Which rules guide your decisions? What would it be like if you could operate on the principles of your Inner Pilot Light instead of your Small Self?

Your Fear Diagnosis

Once you understand how your fears are running the show and where your fears come from, you're ready to firm up your Fear Diagnosis and write it down. Once you've done this, you'll be able to use the information your fears have illuminated to direct you to the tools you need to heal. Call upon Steps 1, 2, and 3 of the Six Steps to Cultivating Courage as you consider this process. If the root causes of your false fears lie in limiting beliefs, go back to Step 1 and get proactive about freeing yourself from the beliefs that hold you back. If lack of aligned support predisposes you to fear, refer to Step 2 and work on building the support you need. If you found it difficult to get to the root causes of your fear, work on Step 3 and let your Inner Pilot Light guide you. If you still feel clueless about where your false fear stems from, see a therapist, work with a spiritual counselor, or seek guidance from someone else skilled in helping you gain insight into what underlies your fear.

COURAGE-CULTIVATING EXERCISE #25

Make Your Own Fear Diagnosis

1. **Ask your Inner Pilot Light, "What lies at the root of my false fears?"**
Pick up a pen and without thinking about it, just write. Let your intuition write your Fear Diagnosis for you. List everything that feels like it could be a cause of unnecessary fear.

2. **If you get stuck, ask yourself the following questions.**
Do any of the Four Fearful Assumptions apply to me?
Are there other limiting beliefs, childhood traumas, or fear-inducing patterns I learned when I was young? Am I burdened by generational fears? If so, what are they?
Am I a pessimist?
Do I lack faith that I can handle whatever comes my way?
Do I need support?
Do I need to serve others?
Am I out of touch with my Inner Pilot Light? Do I lack trust in this guidance?

STEP 5: PRESCRIBE. *Write The Prescription for Courage for yourself.*

Once you've worked on shifting your beliefs, finding the right support, learning to use your intuition to discern true fear from false fear, and diagnosing the root causes of your fear, you may feel inspired to *do* something about it. That's where your Prescription for Courage comes in—but keep in mind that your Prescription for Courage isn't always about "doing something." It might be a silent sabbatical during which you *do nothing.* The Prescription for Courage isn't always about radical movement. Sometimes it's about wild stillness.

In fact, your Prescription for Courage isn't so much an action plan as an opportunity to set intentions and make decisions that might command action. That's why every Prescription for Courage begins the same way, by getting very clear with yourself about your intentions and your readiness. When your intentions are clear and you're really ready to transform your life, you will.

Is Now the Time?

When you are fuzzy on your intentions or try to take action before you're ready, false fears tend to get blown up into big hairy monsters. Then these amplified fears sabotage you, and you feel like you just can't trust yourself to follow through on anything. Maybe you pay big bucks to start a transformational growth program, but you wind up quitting halfway through. You promise yourself you'll start meditating, but every day, you find excuses not to. You look up rehab programs but then you never go. You finally break up with your boyfriend, then two days later, you sleep with him. You try to quit your job, until they offer you a raise and you get sucked in again.

Every time you make a promise to yourself you don't keep, you eat away at your integrity and your courage. Rather than jumping into action, the first step in every Prescription for Courage is to get crystal clear on the change you wish to create. Then wait to take action until you've decided you're *really ready.* Draw the line in the sand. Step over it with every ounce of inner fortitude you've got. Know that this time, it's for real.

If you're not ready, that's okay. Be compassionate with yourself. Don't beat yourself into courage. Trust me, that approach is guaranteed to fail every time. Loving yourself into courageous action works so much better. When you approach courageous action with compassion and self-love, something magical happens. At some point, when you least expect it, a spark catches fire. The flame grows. The light outshines the darkness. And *boom*—you're making brave changes in your life.

When this time comes, it doesn't come as yet another empty resolution. It comes from within, and it feels different from the promises you make and break or the changes you try to implement in order to please other people. One day, you simply care so much about yourself, your health, your happiness, and your commitment to courage that you simply decide *the time is now.*

If you don't feel ready yet, focus on the first four steps until you do. Be patient. You may still be gestating, and as any woman who has ever been pregnant knows, you can't rush gestation. Don't worry that you're not ready yet. Trust that the time will come when you are ripe for change. Be open to action when that time does come.

Are you ready? Is now the time?

The Elements of the Prescription

There's no boilerplate Prescription for Courage everyone can follow, because this process is so deeply personal. But as part of my research, I asked people I considered brave what practices they use to cultivate courage, and some consistent themes emerged. Almost every person I interviewed recommended meditation as an essential foundation to living a more courageous life, and I concur. Courage lives in your spiritual essence, which you can only access in the space between your thoughts. Anything that helps you create space between your thoughts boosts how brave you can be.

Another key factor that came up time and time again in my interviews was trust. Almost all the brave people I interviewed said they had to learn to trust not only themselves and their intuition, but something bigger than themselves. Do you trust that even when times get rough, you'll land butter side up? If you don't already trust that that's so, are you willing to change your mindset? When you start collecting evidence that you *will* always land butter side up, even in the midst of challenges, it becomes easier to trust yourself and the Divine.

Michelle said that when she looked back in retrospect on all of the truly frightening times in her life, she was amazed at how courageous she'd already been. It makes her feel like she can trust herself when she gets scared now. Jen said that it helps to remind herself every day that all is as it should be. She repeats this as a mantra many times each day—*All is as it should be*—and it stops her from following the fearful thoughts in her head. Charlotte repeats a similar mantra—*All will be well*.

In other ways, I found these people's approaches to courage to be as distinct as the individuals themselves. Emilee finds it helpful to acknowledge her fear as a scared inner child. She talks to her scared inner child and reassures her that she is safe. Sam suggests looking at your hand when you feel afraid. When you look at your hand, she explains, it brings you into the present moment and the fear voice stops. Your hand places a gap in the thought stream where peace can come in. Ruth finds heart- and chest-opening yoga poses helpful when she needs to feel brave. She says it's hard to shrink or be small when you are physically lifting and opening your heart.

Sandra, who took up an unusual sport at 47 when she started learning routines on the trampoline, says that if she feels afraid, she reminds herself, "Hey, if I can do a backflip, I can handle [insert current fear]." Anna recommends taking a moment and remembering a time when you felt like you were on top of the world: remember what you were doing, how you were feeling, what was surrounding you, who was with you, the smells, the sounds, the sights, then stand tall and let that moment fill you up with courage. Lottie suggests making a list of all the frightening things you've already done or experienced in your life; acknowledge that you got through these challenges, and use this as evidence to remind yourself how brave and strong you really are.

Books to Change Your Life

Many of the people I interviewed credit certain books as key parts of their Prescriptions for Courage. These books don't necessarily have to be self-help books, books about psychology or spirituality, or religious texts. Books of paintings or photographic images or poetry may inspire your courage. Certainly, my own Prescription for Courage has included hundreds of books, but a few key ones have been so influential for me that they seem worth sharing. The following list includes many books that changed my life, but also some that came up time and time again in my interviews. Of course, the books that change _your_ life may be completely different. Play with engaging your intuition when you peruse the bookstore. Allow the right books to speak to you. Let yourself be drawn to the ones that stand out.

While many people—myself included—draw inspiration from classic spiritual and religious texts, such as the Bible, the Torah, the Koran, the I Ching, the Tao Te Ching, and _A Course in Miracles,_ I've excluded these obviously inspirational books from this list because they're already so widely known. Instead, I've limited this list to nonreligious books I've personally read and can therefore endorse. There are surely many more wonderful books that could change your life. Definitely don't exclude a book that feels like it might resonate with you just because it's not on this list!

These are in no particular order, so don't assume that those higher on the list have been more influential than others.

30 BOOKS THAT COULD CHANGE YOUR LIFE

1. *The Untethered Soul* by Michael A. Singer

2. *Falling into Grace* by Adyashanti

3. *Daring Greatly* by Brené Brown

4. *An Open Heart* by the Dalai Lama

5. *The Power of Now* by Eckhart Tolle

6. *Kitchen Table Wisdom* by Rachel Naomi Remen, M.D.

7. *Finding Your Way in a Wild New World* by Martha Beck, Ph.D.

8. *Outrageous Openness* by Tosha Silver

9. *Broken Open* by Elizabeth Lesser

10. *Man's Search for Meaning* by Viktor E. Frankl

11. *Peace Is Every Step* by Thich Nhat Hanh

12. *The Road Less Traveled* by M. Scott Peck

13. *A Path with Heart* by Jack Kornfield

14. *Be Here Now* by Ram Dass

15. *The Places that Scare You* by Pema Chödrön

16. *Feel the Fear and Do It Anyway* by Susan Jeffers

17. *A Return to Love* by Marianne Williamson

18. *Care of the Soul* by Thomas Moore

19. *My Grandfather's Blessings* by Rachel Naomi Remen, M.D.

20. *The Dark Side of the Light Chasers* by Debbie Ford

21. *Living in the Light* by Shakti Gawain

22. *The Game of Life and How to Play It* by Florence Scovel Shinn

23. *Sacred Contracts* by Caroline Myss

24. *Seat of the Soul* by Gary Zukav

25. *Love Without Conditions* by Paul Ferrini

26. *Loving What Is* by Byron Katie

27. *Tibetan Book of Living and Dying* by Sogyal Rinpoche

28. *The Courage to Heal* by Ellen Bass and Laura Davis

29. *A New Earth* by Eckhart Tolle

30. *I Am That* by Nisargadatta Maharaj

Putting It All Together

In the next exercise, you'll be invited to create your own action plan for cultivating courage. This process is self-guided and requires trusting your intuition. You may find yourself writing things that make no sense to your cognitive mind. Don't question yourself too much. When you overanalyze, your cognitive mind tends to try to talk your intuition out of what it senses. Trust yourself and let your Inner Pilot Light show the way.

COURAGE-CULTIVATING EXERCISE #26

Write Your Prescription for Courage

1. **Get a piece of paper or open a document on your computer, and title it "My Prescription for Courage."** (To download a Prescription Pad for your Prescription for Courage, go to TheFearCureBook.com and register for the free Prescription for Courage Kit.)

2. **State a clear intention, either out loud or in writing.** Why have you undertaken this process? What outcome are you hoping to create? What would "success" look and feel like? Why do you want to be more courageous?

3. **Assess your readiness.** Be honest with yourself. Are you really ready to change? It's okay if you're not. This is a natural gestation process, and there's no need to pressure yourself. If you know what you need to do, but you know you're not quite ready to do it, go ahead and write your Prescription. *You don't have to take any action now.* You can set it aside until the time is right for you to draw that line in the sand and step across it.

4. **Ask yourself, "What do I need in order to cultivate courage?"** Write down anything that comes to mind: a practice you want to start, a class you want to take, a change in your environment, a person you want to call upon for support, a book you want to read, a boundary you want to set, or anything else that comes to mind. It's perfectly fine if your Prescription for Courage lists only one small baby step. That one thing could change everything for you, or it could lead to other actions that will. Don't underestimate the value of taking even one step. If you're not sure what to put on your list, start by ensuring that you have some sort of regular stillness-inducing practice, such as yoga, meditation, qigong, or tai chi. Then move on to considering all the Courage-Cultivating Exercises scattered throughout this book and ask yourself whether you wish to adopt any of these practices. Consider all the Courage-Cultivating Exercises in Part Two. Might any of them

help you shift from the Four Fearful Assumptions to the Four Courage-Cultivating Truths? Consider all the Courage-Cultivating Exercises in Steps 1 through 4 of this chapter. Do you need to implement practices to shift your beliefs? Do you need soul support? Are there practices, programs, or books that might develop your intuition or help you heal your fear from its roots? Check out the 30 Books that Could Change Your Life. Review the 20 Ideas for Cultivating Courage in Appendix B on page 273. See if you get any ideas that light you up. Your Prescription for Courage may be as simple as the decision to find your soul community, and once you feel supported, you may find that you feel braver. For some people, just leaving the house requires radical courage. Don't be afraid to start small, but also know that it's okay to push yourself beyond your comfort zone. See Appendix D if you're curious to read my own personal Prescription for Courage.

5. Start small so you can revel in your success when you bravely act upon an idea you might have been afraid to implement before. Don't forget to celebrate your courage when you do! As you go, keep a list of brave actions you take as your courage grows, and reflect upon it when you need inspiration.

STEP 6: SURRENDER. *Release attachment to outcomes and accept what is.*

We live in a culture that teaches us that if you want something, you have to go get it. Push. Strive. Put your ass in the chair until it's done. Make it happen. Go for it. Put your nose to the grindstone. No pain, no gain. If it's not going well, try harder. But never let 'em see you sweat. And for Pete's sake, don't stop and savor what you've achieved, because there's a bigger goal right around the corner.

These are the principles I was operating from when I was on a flailing book tour in 2010. I had scheduled my book tour ahead of time in many different cities, and I had two other people along with me to help me manage the logistics. But when we got to some of these cities, nothing was actually happening. Because of all the events we anticipated in New York City, we were paying for five nights in an expensive hotel, yet there weren't any actual book tour events set up. I was confused and frustrated. What about all the national media that was supposed to be happening? What about the book signings we had scheduled? The book tour was costing a lot of money, and yet few people were actually buying my books.

I was trying to figure out how to rescue the tour when I reached out to Dr. Christiane Northrup, who offered me this gem of wisdom: "Lissa, you are brilliant at DOING, but you need to learn how to RECEIVE. Be less sperm, more egg."

Christiane recognized that I was in the midst of a dark night of the soul, and while she could have waved her magic wand and rescued me, she wanted to help me learn an important lesson. She e-mailed me, *Lissa, of course you are a do-er. There's no way to get through a surgical residency if you're not. But then, in order to thrive, you'll find that what got you to where you are will kill you if you continue! You're coming upon the developmental stage where the doing will really bite you in the ass if you don't learn to receive.*

When I read this, I got the goose bumps of truth. For years, being "spermy" was an adaptive mechanism for me. It served me well and allowed me to survive 12 years of medical education that gave me many gifts. Now this adaptation no longer served me, and it was time for me to let it go. But how?

Christiane started me down an "eggy" path that led me to Martha Beck, Rachel Naomi Remen, and Tosha Silver, who reinforced this essential spiritual lesson. Being "spermy" can be a highly successful strategy if your goal is world domination via sheer might, ten thousand hours, the force of your will, noble levels of determination, and utter exhaustion. If you're trying to build a business, write a book, achieve a vision, complete a project, or otherwise bring into form something that exists only in your mind, I can personally vouch for the effectiveness of this traditionally masculine approach. I spent about three decades of my life operating in this paradigm of "success," and I'm here to tell you—it can absolutely work. But what I came to realize under the tutelage of my feminine mentors is that there's another way of being in the world, and it's all about surrender.

What does it mean to be "eggy"? Being eggy is all about setting goals but releasing attachment to outcomes. It's about surrendering to what wants to become, rather than pushing for what your ego wants to make happen. It's to put your desires out there, to turn them over to Universal Intelligence, and to trust that whatever happens is in the highest good. Being eggy requires trusting that it's a purposeful universe, and even if things aren't going the way you hoped, it's all happening for some reason that you may never quite understand.

It's easy to misconstrue this feminine principle. Being eggy isn't about being passive or lacking ambition; it's about trusting that when you move in the direction of joy, ease, peace, harmony, and love, and when you let go of attachment to outcomes, the Universe falls over itself trying to bring about your highest good. When you surrender the grasping, you make room for that which you desire to come to you if it's aligned with the highest good.

Being eggy certainly isn't hard. It's effortless, really. But this way of being doesn't feel easy to the ego, because it requires managing the anxiety that comes with not pushing, striving, and overworking. It also commands you to align with your integrity, and this may require you to do things that feel very risky, like saying no to people you love or setting clear boundaries at work.

Tosha Silver teaches that, while there are similarities, being eggy is not about the "law of attraction" the way it is taught in many popular New Age books. It's not about making a laundry list of your ego's desires and then visualizing, affirming, and manifesting your patootie off. So many people I interviewed about fear confessed to being frustrated with the law of attraction. They'd spent four years trying to visualize, affirm, and attract a Ferrari, yet they were still stuck taking the bus! They had made a dozen vision boards, posted affirmations on the refrigerator, watched the Ferrari like a movie in their mind, and felt the wind in their hair as they saw themselves driving down Highway 1. But there was still no Ferrari. This is not what being eggy is all about. It's just a whole other way to be spermy. Being eggy is about surrendering your desires, rather than attaching to your longing.

Surrendering desire, will, control, and the inclination to over-work is the most unnatural thing in the world for me. Some people I've met are the opposite—they err on the side of being too eggy. They decide to become life coaches, undergo life coach training, turn over their desire for clients to Divine Will, and then sit back waiting for clients to show up, without ever putting up a website or announcing that they're looking for clients on social media or via e-mail. But most people in our culture—men and women alike—trend toward the spermy.

The eggy way of operating may not always get you what you want if what you desire is purely materialistic or focused solely on your personal gain. I'm not suggesting that there's anything wrong with desiring material things. Surely, there's not. It's just that when you turn over your Small Self's desires and trust the direction of the highest good, you'll be surprised how something beyond what your Small Self can attach to can begin to occur.

Surrendering into Courage

When you take courageous action in service to the greater good, you can do it the spermy way or you can choose to be eggy instead. Don't get me wrong. The spermy path can be very "successful." It's just that it isn't always fulfilling. You may very well achieve everything your ego desires, only to discover that achieving your ego's desires doesn't satisfy your soul. Maybe you get rich and famous and hook up with your dream date. But is it making you happy? Do you feel deeply enriched, connected, and at peace? Are you free from the prison of false fear? Or do you now feel afraid of losing it all? Do you pressure yourself to go get even more? Do you trade one set of false fears for another?

While being spermy may be an effective adaptation when you're trying to make it through grad school or plow through the pile of papers on your desk at work, there are ways in which being spermy doesn't work at all. You can't sperm your child into growing up happy. You can't sperm your way out of cancer. You can't sperm your way to the love of your life. Sure, you read parenting books, eat a healthy cancer-fighting diet, and get on Match.com, but no amount of striving will achieve these desires.

And you can't sperm your way to courage. That's where Step 6 comes in. You can do everything within your power to become more brave. You can work on shifting your beliefs, finding support for your soul, tapping into your intuition, diagnosing the root causes of your false fears, and writing and implementing your Prescription for Courage. You can practice every exercise in this book and read every book on the list I've shared with you. You can meditate, take workshops, go to conferences, practice yoga, and move into an ashram. But you can't force yourself to be brave.

In the Bible, Philippians 4:6 says, "Don't worry about anything; instead, pray about everything." Regardless of your religious inclinations, prayer has the power to release fear. Whenever you notice fear slipping in, convert your fearful thoughts into offerings of surrender. Sound too simple? Or too hard? Tosha Silver would recommend saying what she calls a "Change Me Prayer," something like "Change me into someone who can let the Divine take the lead."

Of course, it's all well and good to talk about surrender in this way, but it's only lip service unless you're able to put it into practice when things get really hard. As I was writing this chapter, my husband and I were in the middle of divorce mediation, and although things started out amicably, I watched two people who care about each other start volleying for position as we talked about how we would divide up our assets. My Small Self had an inner tantrum that boiled down to *Mine, mine, MINE. I'm scared of losing everything I've worked so hard to earn. I have to protect myself—NOW.* I found myself slipping into fearful self-protection mode without considering what was best for this man I've loved for 12 years.

I wrote to Tosha and told her I was trying to surrender the entire divorce to Divine Will, but I was having a hard time. She replied, *Here's what works for folks who are divorcing. Just say, "One hundred percent of the money belongs to God, and God has the perfect solution." Ask to be shown the perfect settlement, as the steward of but not the owner of the money. It makes a world of difference. Once it's offered 100 percent to the Divine, the right actions become clear. Don't misunderstand; surrender has nothing to do with being passive. You will simply be shown what to do with the assets that belong to God and always have.*

You'll feel like you dropped a hundred pounds when you let this go, she went on. *You are ready, Lissa. This is the graduate school of surrender. You can do this.*

I wrote back: *Yes, I'm ready. I'm really, really, really ready. But I don't know if I'm strong enough to do this. I do think of all these things as "mine." It's amazing how this divorce process feeds the righteousness and judgment of the Small Self. I'm thinking the most horrible things about this man I've loved for years.*

Tosha replied: *Don't beat up your Small Self for its tantrum. That's what our Small Selves do! Just give that scared little kid a hug. Stop "trying" to surrender through the Small Self. It won't know how. Let God do it instead.*

I accepted the invitation and said a Change Me prayer: "Change Me into someone who can surrender this to Divine Will." The minute I said it, I felt a jolt of electricity zip up my spine. My whole body got goose bumps, and my heart felt full of peace.

Don't get me wrong—it still wasn't easy for me. The chatter in my head told me that it's not safe to surrender, that I might get screwed, that I needed to control this divorce and steer it toward my own interests instead. But that's how tenacious the Small Self can be. When it senses that you're on the brink of really letting the courage of your Inner Pilot Light take the lead, it will pull out all the stops to convince you how much you need it to be in charge.

I'm scared as I write this. I feel like I'm jumping into the vast abyss and I'm afraid I won't get what I want if I let go. But I don't want to let my fear run the show anymore. I'm going to feel afraid and leap anyway. Tosha's right. I'm ready. The question is—are you?

Arguably, surrender is the most important of the Six Steps to Cultivating Courage. When you master the art of surrender, you come into right relationship with uncertainty, develop a healthy relationship with your desires, watch your fear dissipate, and become naturally brave. You no longer depend on fear to keep you safe, because you trust that something bigger than you is on it already. Then you can let go of the safety bar and make yourself a vessel in service to the highest good.

It's hard to break this all down into some "how to" process, but in case you need help learning to surrender, I've distilled several steps from the teachings of my spiritual advisors in order to help you call in your courage. Most of these lessons in surrender draw upon Tosha Silver's teachings from *Outrageous Openness,* as well as Martha Beck's "Four Technologies of Magic" from *Finding Your Way in a Brave New World.*

Courage-Cultivating Exercise #27

Practice Surrender

1. **Name Your Desire**
   Whether you're applying this process to your desire to be less afraid, your desire to get healthy, or your desire to find love, the process of surrender begins the same way. In spite of what you might have been taught in Sunday school, desire is never wrong. It's a signpost pointing toward what lights you up, feeds your soul, sparks your enthusiasm, and makes you feel alive. Sometimes we're misguided in what we think we desire. You might think you want your best friend's husband, but what you really want is the kind of soulful connection you feel when you're with him—which you're likely to find in someone else in a way that doesn't threaten your integrity and lead you into betraying your best friend. Desire is simply information. It's feedback about what sparks your Inner Pilot Light.

2. **Offer Your Desire**
   The minute you identify your desire, offer it over to the Divine. Want to become brave? Offer it over. Afraid your husband is cheating on you? Offer it. Worried you'll pick the wrong gift for your bestie's birthday? Make an offering. Frustrated from trying to fix the computer glitch that just ate your blog

post? Surrender it to the Divine. Usually, in our culture, we skip this step—or come to it on our knees, as a last resort, when everything else we know how to do has failed—but really it's the first thing we should do.

How do you offer up a desire? The Small Self will always try to take control of the process. But that's not what the act of surrender is about. It's not about teaching your Small Self how to surrender so you can get what you want. It's about making an offering to the Divine and being genuinely willing to accept whatever is in the highest good, even if it flies in the face of what you desire. Offering is about unburdening yourself from the weight of your longing. Tosha Silver teaches us to see the desire like a 100-pound box pushing heavily on the heart. Visualize this, then visualize giving the weighty box to whatever Higher Power feels right to you. The longing is no longer yours to force into being. The problem is no longer yours to solve. Tosha also teaches what she calls "Change Me" prayers, because they bypass the attachment of the Small Self. For example, "Change me into someone who can surrender instead of someone who has to always be in control."

As Martha Beck says, "Attention. Intention. No tension." The key is releasing attachment to the specific outcome you desire. Let your prayer be "This—or better." Be open to miracles.

3. **Get Wordless**
This is an energetic step, which requires dropping into a certain state of consciousness. Getting Wordless, which activates both sides of your brain, is what Martha Beck calls the "First Technology of Magic." Jung called this Wordless state the "collective unconscious," and Martha likens it to tapping into some sort of "energy internet" that allows you to hook into something larger than little ol' you. Getting Wordless can be facilitated by techniques such as feeling into the insides of your hands, pulling your senses into "open focus," following your own bloodstream, "sense-drenching" (letting yourself experience the world through all five senses at once), connecting deeply with nature, sacred dance, unfocusing your eyes and thinking about sleep, or

opening the mind through the use of paradox. For specific instructions on how to practice these techniques, read Martha's book.

4. **Tap into Oneness**
    Tapping into Oneness (Martha's "Second Technology of Magic") is about getting out of the Small Self and becoming One with all that is—allowing the separation between you, other life forms, and what you desire to dissolve. When this happens, it's as if you're sending an e-mail on the energy internet, bringing the essence of what you desire closer to you. Don't forget that what gets closer may not be the thing you thought you desired. It may be a feeling state you think you'll get when you have a certain thing. Perhaps you think you want a million dollars, but what you really desire is the feeling of ease that accompanies your idea of having a million dollars. It may be that ease shows up in other ways, minus the money.
    Some of Martha's techniques for tapping into Oneness include easefully bending flatware by energetically becoming One with it and feeling it "melt" under your hands, letting the produce in the grocery store communicate with you about which plants are good for you and which ones aren't, entraining other humans into a calm state of consciousness, or telepathically communicating with your pet—or even a wild animal—and seeing if it responds to you.

5. **Imagine Your Intention into Being**
    Imagining yourself being brave represents Martha's "Third Technology of Magic." Although it may seem similar to fantasizing, this process is vastly different. Fantasy has a quality of grasping about it. It almost hurts to fantasize because you're afraid you'll be disappointed if you don't get what you're dreaming of. Fantasy often has an unachievable feel about it; Imagining feels as though, in some dimension, what you desire has already come to be. Imagining is about sensing what yearns to be created, rather than merely getting what you want.
    Here's an example. Dennis, my friend whose stories you have heard throughout this book, is Dutch. At the time I was writing this, he had been living in the United States for 18 months, and his attorney

advised him against applying for the green card he had been counting on in order to stay in California. Unless something changed, Dennis would have to leave the United States in a few weeks. This was not what he desired. To his rational mind, staying in California was what was best for him. But when Dennis shifted his consciousness by going Wordless and tapping into Oneness, and then started Imagining, he saw himself doing something quite different—going to Peru to study with shamans for a while, then coming back to California with permission to stay. Although he didn't consciously want to leave California at all, that feeling of "rightness" about going first to Peru began growing stronger in Dennis. He was seeing pictures of himself going to Peru. This is how Imagining works. By opening himself to sensing what wanted to become, Dennis started co-creating something. Would he get the right visa to stay in the U.S.? Would he go to Peru? Would he get a green card? No way to say for sure. But by Imagining the possible outcomes, he was participating in the creation of what was unfolding energetically. The same can be true for you when you Imagine yourself taking courageous action.*

6. **Be on the Alert for Guidance**
Now that you've gotten clear on your desire, turned it over to the Universe, practiced Wordlessness and Oneness, and Imagined what you desire coming into being, it's time to let yourself be guided. Practice radical listening. Watch for signs from the Universe. Pay attention to your intuitive knowing. The signs are everywhere, and they're trying to get your attention, but you'll miss them if you're not on the

---

*   In case you're curious about what happened to Dennis, his visa did not come through, so he moved to Peru for six months, intent upon committing to his spiritual growth. I went to meet him there, and we journeyed together up to 16,000 feet in the Andes, where we stayed in an indigenous Q'eros village with the local shamans, studying the healing modalities and spiritual teachings of these wise beings. Dennis subsequently underwent shamanic training and was initiated into his new calling. We now teach together about letting fear cure you, surrendering to Divine Will, and other aspects of spiritual healing. Although Dennis's Small Self did not initially get what it wanted, his soul clearly got what it yearned for.

lookout. Anticipate guidance and then tune in. Be aware of the tendency to misinterpret guidance, especially when it is guiding you away from what you desire. This is where nonattachment is especially crucial. Remember, it's not about getting what you want; it's about surrendering and aligning with what wants to become.

7. **Take Inspired Action**
When you're paying attention to guidance, at some point you will be called to DO SOMETHING. Martha's "Fourth Technology of Magic" defines this stage as "Forming." Tosha Silver suggests paying attention to *spanda* at this point in the process. *Spanda* is a Sanskrit term that means "to move a little." In other words, surrendering doesn't equal passivity. Sometimes you'll be called to inspired action. Can't tell whether or not to act? Then use your body as a compass. If you're considering taking some action in the direction of your desire, do you feel a full-body YES that makes you leap up with enthusiasm? Or does it feel like a "should" that leaves your body exhausted at the mere thought of it? Inspired action feels energizing and easeful, while ego-driven striving can leave you feeling drained, stressed, or overwhelmed with dread. Inspired action may require you to put your butt in the chair and do something challenging, but it will still have the feeling of play about it.

8. **Be Patient**
This is the hard part. You may wish you could become brave overnight. You may wish you suddenly had what it takes to ditch false fear and let courage take the lead in all your decision making. But sometimes what you desire doesn't show up exactly when you want it in exactly the form you want it in. This is when people have a tendency to get frustrated, blame themselves for not "manifesting" correctly, or get angry at God for not delivering the desire on a silver platter. Once you've practiced the other steps, be willing to wait. And wait. And wait. Trust divine timing. And be willing to change course if guidance leads you to do so.

9. **Practice Gratitude**
   Maybe you got what you desired and fear is a thing
   of the past for you. But maybe, if you're like most
   mere mortals, you're still afraid from time to time.
   Either way, find the perfection in it. Be grateful
   for the learning. If your desire came into being, let
   yourself be awash in the grace of it all. If it didn't,
   be grateful that something even better—whatever
   wants to become—is on its way. Even if you only feel
   a little more brave at the end of this journey, express
   thanks.

   As Mama Gena says, "Unexpressed blessings
   turn to shit." Thank your courage—or whatever else
   you may have called into being. Trust the process.
   Lather. Rinse. Repeat.

When I first took a workshop with Tosha to learn tools for living a more eggy life, I had an epiphany. With a wrinkled brow, I approached Tosha after the workshop, and I told her that in *Mind Over Medicine,* I had written Six Steps to Healing Yourself, but I wondered whether I had written them in the wrong order. The six steps in *Mind Over Medicine* are the same steps as those in this book—BELIEVE, SUPPORT, INTUITION, DIAGNOSE, PRESCRIBE, and SURRENDER. In *Mind Over Medicine,* I wrote about the importance of surrender, turning your illness over to Divine Will, and letting go of attachment to outcomes. But I made surrender Step 6.

"Tosha," I said, sheepishly. "Surrender should be Step One."

Tosha nodded. "Yes, darling. Surrender is always Step One."

It's the truth. Life is easier and less frightening if surrender is always Step 1. But in this process, because I suspect many of you are like me, I've kept SURRENDER as Step 6, not because I don't believe it's possible to turn over our desires first thing, but because most of us feel comfortable doing everything else we possibly can first. Then, often on our knees, we'll let go.

Many seekers approach the act of surrender this way. First, you do everything within your power to get what you want. If fear is making you sick or miserable, you'll probably be motivated to do everything you can with sheer might, determination, and will. You'll meditate. You'll find your soul community. You'll practice heightening your intuition. You'll work on your limiting beliefs. Then, if you've tried everything and you're still feeling burdened by the suffering that accompanies false fear, you may finally be willing to fall on your knees and surrender.

Surrender in this form is often an act of helpless desperation. But it need not be this way. If you're willing to turn over your fears to a Higher Power early on, you just might find that courage runs right up to you and jumps into your heart.

You don't have to start with the big guns from the get-go. You can start practicing surrender in small ways. Looking for the right parking spot? Surrender. Hoping for a seat on an oversold flight? Surrender. Wishing your boss would let you go home early on Friday? Surrender. Pick little things and practice surrendering what you desire. Pay attention to what happens. Keep your eyes, ears, and heart open. Look for signs. Trust the guidance that shows up. Then be brave enough to let the guidance direct your decisions. When we learn to surrender, the feminine principle weaves its way into our lives and changes how we operate, not just as individuals, but as a culture.

For centuries, modern culture has been dominated by the masculine principle. In many ways, this has been a blessing. The masculine principle has gotten us far. We can cure many cancers because of the masculine principle. We've extended our life expectancy by 30 years in the past century because of the masculine principle. The Internet exists because of the masculine principle. We made it into outer space because of the masculine principle. The drive to explore, innovate, and push the envelope has served us in countless ways. The masculine principle can be a powerful and healthy force for change, innovation, and forward motion.

But many of the systems within our culture have been corrupted by the destructive, profane version of this force. The health care system, the legal system, the education system, the banking system, corporate culture—these have been overtaken with greed, competition, and the self-absorbed motives of those in power. We've lost touch with what it means to cooperate, open our hearts, compromise, and collaborate. We need a shift in the direction of the feminine to bring our culture back into balance.

The surrender being asked of you in Step 6 is an invitation to allow the feminine principle to balance out your life too. All change is a dance between making it happen and letting it happen. That's what the Six Steps to Cultivating Courage are all about.

TAKE THE FIRST STEP

There's a wonderful line often attributed to Anaïs Nin: "And the time came when the risk to remain tight in a bud was more painful than the risk it took to blossom." I understand that the risk it takes to blossom takes a lot of courage. This is your invitation. What will it take for your longing to awaken to outweigh your fear of the unknown? What will it take for you to find the courage to blossom? You may have picked up this book because you struggle with fear, but in spite of what you may think, you are already impossibly brave. A worried, anxious, and fearful part of you limits you, but an infinitely greater part of you radiates courage. You already have the power to access this inner strength, but what you've learned in this book will strengthen your relationship with it and bring it even more within your reach.

In spite of what you may think, *you are not in control of your life*. This is not meant to frighten you. It's meant to liberate you. You are not at the mercy of a random, chaotic universe flouncing you around like a yo-yo on a string. This is not a dangerous world always threatening to hurt you. It's a purposeful universe that offers you opportunities for soul growth that may arise in the form of both delight and adversity. Rather than resisting adversity when it appears, you can lean in and know that you are learning and you are not only safe; you are loved. You may not understand what your soul is learning right away. You may feel victimized. Life might seem unfair. It's only natural to feel this way. But when you look back, you will see that it all makes sense, that even times of tragedy were filled with purpose, and that your soul grew even as you grieved.

I know how you yearn for certainty. I do too. It's only human. We all long to know that everything we cherish will last forever and nothing we fear will ever come to pass. But we forget that by guarding against uncertainty, we close ourselves off to possibility. When we don't know what the future holds, ANYTHING IS POSSIBLE. When we welcome in mystery, awe and wonder might walk in with it.

Don't let your fear limit you, dear reader. Let it wake you up instead. Invite it to hand you the key that opens the soul cage and sets you free. As long as you require certainty, you won't take risks, and you have to take risks if you want to know joy. You must risk your heart. You must risk loss. You must be willing to experience pain in order to realize your full potential—who you really are. This requires radical courage. You will be asked to stand in a rush of love so potent that you can barely breathe; yet, in that moment, you will be overwhelmed with how vulnerable you are. To learn to be that vulnerable, to leave your heart that open, is the ultimate life test. There's no limit to the number of times you can retake this test. No one cares whether you pass or fail the test. You can let courage take the wheel or you can let fear lead. Nobody will judge you either way.

But as a doctor who has been at the bedsides of a lot of dying people, I can vouch for the fact that the dying rarely regret not having enough control over their lives. They regret that they didn't risk more. They regret dreams they didn't pursue, passions they squandered. But even more, they regret not opening their hearts all the way. They regret love unspoken, ways in which they held back, the armor they wore in order to protect themselves in their vulnerability.

Please don't be one of those people who dies with regret. Don't let fear hold you back. It's not too late. There's still time. Instead of being limited by your fears, you can let the brave part of you take the wheel for the rest of your life. You can be one of those people who dies spent, with no passion unfulfilled and no love unexpressed, full of the inner stillness that comes from alignment with your true self. Your heart is this capacious. Your brave is as big as the ocean. You have no idea how vast you are.

You can start right now. You hold within you the power to shift everything in an instant. Your true self yearns to break free and bless the world.

Martin Luther King, Jr., said, "Faith is taking the first step even when you don't see the whole staircase." You will know it is finally time to blossom when the pain of staying put and your yearning for courage exceed your fear of change. If you're ready, dear one, take the first step.

APPENDIX A

13 Techniques for Shifting Beliefs

1. **Byron Katie's "The Work."** This technique is very effective at identifying and shifting limiting beliefs. Read Byron Katie's book *Loving What Is,* sign up for one of her workshops, fill out one of the "Judge Your Neighbor" worksheets at TheWork.com, or see a therapist or coach trained in her technique.

2. **Cognitive-Behavioral Therapy (CBT).** A common psychotherapeutic approach practiced by many therapists, cognitive-behavioral therapy is problem-focused and action-oriented. CBT addresses dysfunctional emotions, self-sabotaging behaviors, and maladaptive cognitive processes through goal-oriented procedures. CBT techniques can help you challenge limiting beliefs and patterns and replace errors in thinking with healthier thoughts meant to decrease emotional distress and self-sabotaging behaviors.

3. **Hypnotherapy.** Hypnotherapy is a form of psychotherapy used to shift thoughts and behaviors at the level of the subconscious mind. Since we operate from the conscious mind only 5 percent of

the time, hypnotherapy can quickly effect change at a deeper level.

4. **Eye Movement Desensitization and Reprocessing (EMDR).** EMDR is a psychotherapeutic technique used for individuals with unresolved trauma. An eight-step protocol guides clients through recalling distressing images while receiving bilateral sensory input, such as side-to-side eye movements or alternating hand taps or auditory tones. EMDR has been proven to help clients process traumatic memories, reduce the consequences of their lingering effects, and improve coping skills.

5. **Psychological Kinesiology (Psych-K).** Psych-K combines positive psychology and kinesiology as a method of communicating directly with the subconscious mind in order to identify and shift limiting beliefs that retard the healing process. By combining affirmations with physical movement, Psych-K activates a whole brain state, which puts the brain in a receptive state for shifting belief.

6. **Emotional Freedom Technique (EFT or Tapping).** EFT is a technique that combines positive psychology with acupressure techniques derived from Chinese medicine. It also has roots in neuro-linguistic programming (NLP), energy medicine, and Thought Field Therapy. As you tap your fingers along acupressure points while releasing negative beliefs and replacing them with positive affirmations, EFT calms the amygdala, reduces fear, and can be effective in shifting belief.

7. **Neuro-Linguistic Programming (NLP).** NLP is based on the interconnection between neurology (neuro), language (linguistic), and how language and the mind interact to affect the body and behavior (programming). NLP is based on the premise

that how we choose our words reflects our inner, subconscious beliefs, and by changing our words, we can shift belief and heal problem areas in our lives.

8. **Whole Body Intelligence.** Steve Sisgold's Whole Body Intelligence uses the body to identify and heal limiting beliefs. Using body awareness to identify how negative beliefs get lodged in the body, Whole Body Intelligence uses a combination of affirmations, movement, somatic awareness, and breath work to release limiting beliefs and change behavior.

9. **Energy/spiritual healing practices.** Many types of energy healing, shamanic healing, or other spiritual healing practices, such as Reiki, Theta healing, faith healing, and intuitive healing, can be useful in addressing limiting beliefs.

10. **Prayer.** Prayer and intention setting can be effective tools for shifting belief. Tosha Silver teaches a form of prayer she calls a "Change Me Prayer." For example, "Change me into someone who isn't afraid." For more on how to surrender and formulate Change Me Prayers, see Courage-Cultivating Exercise #27.

11. **Breathing techniques.** A variety of breath work modalities, such as those used in some meditation or yoga practices, can be utilized to alter negative thought patterns.

12. **Affirmations.** With enough repetition, positive affirmations such as "I am courageous" or "I trust my intuition" can replace negative beliefs in the subconscious mind. Post these affirmations around your house and repeat them when you first wake up in the morning, as well as just before you go to bed. Make them your mantras during meditation. Record them and play them on your phone or MP3 player. In order for affirmations to be effective, they need

to become second nature, so they become imprinted upon the subconscious mind.

13. **Avoidance.** Exposure to fear-inducing influences, such as watching the news, reading the newspaper, viewing scary movies, or spending a lot of time with others who are fearful can influence your beliefs. Especially when you are in a vulnerable transition state, trying to shift your own beliefs, you may find it helpful to create a cocoon that protects you from unnecessarily fearful influences. Once you've made it through your gestation phase, you'll be less vulnerable, but at least in the beginning, you may want to stay in your faith bubble.

APPENDIX B

20 Ideas for Cultivating Courage

1. See a therapist, hire a life coach, or develop a relationship with a spiritual teacher.

2. Sign up for a transformational growth workshop or program (such as Hoffman Institute, Landmark Forum, or a men's or women's workshop).

3. Start a meditation practice.

4. Train for a race.

5. Embark upon a travel quest.

6. Volunteer.

7. Go on a retreat (try Esalen Institute, Omega Institute, or Kripalu).

8. Pursue a pilgrimage (walking the Camino de Santiago or the Pacific Crest Trail).

9. Commit to a movement practice (yoga, Zumba, Nia, Journey Dance, Soul Motion, 5Rhythms).

10. Pick up a new hobby.

11. Take a self-defense class (martial arts, kickboxing, domestic violence protection classes).

12. Learn a new skill (a foreign language, an art form, playing an instrument, interior decorating, writing).

13. Push the limits of your sexuality (S Factor, Tantra, reading erotica, experimenting with sex toys).

14. Treat yourself to radical self-care (indulge in baths, read a book just for fun, go to a spa, get a massage, paint your nails, take a whole day to yourself).

15. Radically change your diet (vegan diet, raw foods, green juice cleansing, superfoods). Or if you're already a health food nut, try cheating!

16. Adopt a rescue pet.

17. Initiate inspiring conversations with strangers.

18. Change your appearance (dye or cut your hair, get a makeover or a tattoo, hire a stylist to help you find your updated look).

19. Commit to recovery (admit to an addiction, sign up for rehab, join a 12-step program).

20. Become One with nature (visit national parks, start gardening, start hiking daily).

APPENDIX C

7 Steps for Creating Your Tribe

Anne Davin, Ph.D., once lived among a Native American tribe and has a special interest in tribe building in modern life. She offers the following guidance, adapted from the Medicine for the Soul teleclass, for finding your soul tribe.

1. **Say yes to every invitation, no matter what.** You never know where your tribe will be. Recognize that each invitation is an aperture to the holy that is seeking to include you in the divine design of life. For this reason, the likelihood that you will encounter soul connections by showing up every time life invites you out into community is very high. Say yes, especially when you really want to say no.

2. **Help others the same amount that you care for yourself.** Operate from the tribal perspective. Rather than focusing on "What can I get?" ask "What can I give?" The getting is in the giving. Hold the door for a stranger. Offer to give directions to someone who is lost. Look for ways to serve every day. Most importantly, give what you most wish to receive.

3. **Go directly into community by choosing one that is already organized around something that turns you on.** This is the quickest way to find like-minded people. Tribal members recognize that groups that have already self-organized are "homes" waiting for them. Make yourself an insider by acting as if you belong. Assume your place is waiting for you.

4. **Ask yourself, *What is my greatest emotional wound?* Then go serve it.** What is the thing that stands most between you and a sense of connection to others? Is it the abuse you suffered as a child? Is it violence at the hands of a battering spouse or the alcoholism of a parent? Go volunteer as a Big Brother or Big Sister, at the battered women's shelter, or at your local halfway house. Use the thing that shattered your trust in life as your means to re-establish trust and connection.

5. **Go on walkabout.** Look at who and what has been pushed to the edges of your world and go on an adventure into those borderlands. To go on modern walkabout, you must first ask, "What is invisible in my world? Are there children in my life? The elderly? What about people who aren't my color or race or age or gender or political persuasion?" List five adjectives that describe you, then reverse them: are people with *these* qualities in your life? Step outside your comfort zone and head out into the unknown as an observer. Allow yourself to get "remade" by the encounter.

6. **Use play as a portal.** When you are at play, relaxed and open, you are most likely to have magical encounters because you are more present to the moment. Take advantage of this. Is your pleasure music? Literature? Flying kites? Running or another physical activity? The whole point is to connect with others in a way that feels authentic. Prioritize your

pleasure and play on a daily basis. Do it with the same commitment you give to brushing your teeth.

7. **Light your own village fire.** What do you love? What breaks you open to awe and wonder? Actively seek out others who share your passion and create opportunities to do it together. Start a book club or a meditation circle. How about bowling? Maybe you love day hikes or cooking. Perhaps your passion lives in serving something or someone else. What magnetizes a tribe is the shared love of its members. Start your own tribe and watch the magic unfold.

APPENDIX D

Lissa's Personal Prescription for Courage

To find the courage to leave conventional medicine in order to pursue my true purpose, sell my house and liquidate my retirement account in order to finance my dream of launching a whole new kind of business, go into debt in order to hire employees so I could grow my fledgling business, and end a marriage that wasn't making me happy, I had to put into practice my own Prescription for Courage. Your transformation is unlikely to consist of life changes as extreme as mine, but the kinds of practices that boost courage tend to be helpful regardless of what you're mustering up the moxie to change.

- Get out of the big city and move from San Diego to a small town on the Northern California coast in order to be surrounded by nature, which helps me feel connected to the Divine and makes me feel braver.

- Begin a daily sitting meditation practice of at least 20 minutes per day, which includes a variety of meditation techniques, devotional practices, and prayer.

- Hike out in nature as often as possible.

- Practice visualizing a "faith bubble" around me to protect myself from all the fears of other people that are being projected onto me (usually under the guise of "protecting me") as I make radical life choices.

- Attract, cultivate, and prioritize people who are actively trying to live an Inner-Pilot-Light-driven life, rather than a Small-Self-driven one. Ask these people for help when my Small Self feels scared.

- Set boundaries and limit time spent with those who are committed to indulging the Small Self.

- Write a blog about being "unapologetically ME" to heal myself from my fear of being perceived as imperfect.

- Without traumatizing myself, challenge myself to try things that scare me as a sort of desensitization therapy. For example, traveling solo to foreign countries, riding roller coasters, and doing ropes courses are all scary to me, but the more I desensitize myself, the less scary they become.

- Make a courage-cultivating home altar filled with meaningful objects that make me feel brave. I use this altar as a place for meditation, intention setting, and the practice of surrender.

- Practice yoga several times per week.

- Purify my body, mind, and spirit with a green juice cleanse, developed by Tricia Barrett, every three months. (For instructions on how to do this yourself, see the Resources section.)

- Listen to music that uplifts my Inner Pilot Light, including Karen Drucker, Snatam Kaur, Deva Premal, Rafael Bejarano, Christine Tulis, Michael Franti, classical music, and the "Inner Pilot Light playlist" I made of songs that touch my soul.

- Attend spiritually based dance workshops such as Nia, Soul Motion, 5Rhythms, Journey Dance, and S Factor.

- Gather with my 5Rhythms ecstatic dance soul community on Sundays.

- Meet monthly with a community of like-minded physicians in a "Finding Meaning in Medicine" study group led by Rachel Naomi Remen.

- Attend dharma talks at Green Gulch Zen Center.

- Make peace with my money fears via books, programs, and one-on-one counseling with Overcoming Underearning coach Barbara Stanny.

- When fears, desires, problems, or adversity arise, practice the art of surrender as described in Step 6 of the Six Steps to Cultivating Courage.

- Read Inner-Pilot-Light-igniting books like the ones listed on pages 249 and 250.

- Listen to teleclasses such as Craig Hamilton's Integral Enlightenment.

- Seek spiritual guidance from a variety of spiritual advisors I trust, including Rachel Naomi Remen, Martha Beck, Tosha Silver, Anne Davin, Elisabeth Manning, Sarah Drew, Sera Beak, Christine Hassler, Jon Rasmussen, Linda Rose, Craig Hamilton, Dennis Couwenberg, and April Sweazy.

- Participate in a monthly spiritual mastermind ("Spiritmind") group with Amy Ahlers, Mike Robbins, Steve Sisgold, and Christine Arylo.

- Attend workshops with spiritual teachers Adyashanti, Tosha Silver, Byron Katie, and Rachel Naomi Remen.

- Attend Martha Beck's African STAR retreat and practice the techniques described in Martha's book *Finding Your Way in a Wild New World* as a way to collect evidence that it's a purposeful universe and we are all One.

- Practice saying no to everything that isn't 100 percent aligned with my Inner Pilot Light, even when it terrifies me to choose soul alignment over security and comfort.

- Whenever fears and doubts arise, practice "being the witness," as described in Courage-Cultivating Exercise #6.

- Avoid fear-inducing news media.

- Pray for spiritual guidance and courage when my Small Self feels scared.

- Whenever I feel frightened, let my Inner Pilot Light nurture my Small Self, as described in Courage-Cultivating Exercise #1.

- Practice acts of radical self-care to soothe my Small Self when it gets scared. Some of my favorite self-soothing techniques are warm baths, foot rubs, aromatherapy, sitting by the ocean, my homemade raw chocolate, lighting candles and incense, dancing by myself, and singing in the shower.

- Write the Daily Flame, daily love letters from your Inner Pilot Light to your Small Self. The practice of writing this daily e-mail as an act of service has helped me learn to identify with this wise, loving voice within me.

RESOURCES

Download the free Prescription for Courage Kit at TheFearCure Book.com.

Learn more about the Whole Health Medicine Institute Physician Training and Health Care Provider training at WholeHealth MedicineInstitute.com.

Learn more about the Medicine for the Soul teleclass program with Lissa Rankin and Rachel Naomi Remen at MedicineForThe SoulRx.com.

Learn more about the Coming Home to Your Spirit teleclass program with Lissa Rankin and Martha Beck at ComingHomeToYour Spirit.com.

Learn more about the Find Your Calling teleclass program with Lissa Rankin, Martha Beck, and Amy Ahlers at FindYourCalling Now.com.

Learn more about the Visionary Ignition Switch teleclass program with Lissa Rankin and Amy Ahlers at VisionaryIgnitionSwitch .com.

Learn more about the green juice cleanse Lissa does every three months at JuiceDietCleanse.com.

Sign up for the Daily Flame, messages from your Inner Pilot Light, at InnerPilotLight.com.

Follow Lissa's blog at LissaRankin.com.

Follow Lissa on Facebook at facebook.com/LissaRankin.

Follow Lissa on Twitter at twitter.com/LissaRankin.

ENDNOTES

Chapter 1

1. Walter B. Cannon, *Bodily Changes in Pain, Hunger, Fear and Rage: An Account of Recent Researches into the Function of Emotional Excitement* (D. Appleton and Company: New York and London, 1927); Hans Selye, "The General Adaptation Syndrome and the Diseases of Adaptation," *The Journal of Clinical Endocrinology & Metabolism* 6, no. 2 (1946): 117–230.

2. "Any Mood Disorder Among Adults," National Institute of Mental Health: http://www.nimh.nih.gov/statistics/1ANYMOODDIS_ADULT.shtml.

3. Hans-Ulrich Wittchen et al., "DSM-III-R Generalized Anxiety Disorder in the National Comorbidity Survey," *Archives of General Psychiatry* 51, no. 5 (May 1994): 355–364.

4. Kendra Cherry, "10 Common Phobias," About.com: http://psychology.about.com/od/phobias/p/commonphobias.htm.

5. Lisa Fritscher, "What Is the Fear of Phobias?," About.com, updated September 3, 2013: http://phobias.about.com/od/phobiaslist/f/What-Is-The-Fear-Of-Phobias.htm.

Chapter 2

1. George L. Engel, "Sudden and Rapid Death During Psychological Stress: Folklore or Folk Wisdom?," *Annals of Internal Medicine* 74, no. 5 (May 1971): 771–782.

2. Jeremy D. Kark, Sylvie Goldman, and Leon Epstein, "Iraqi Missile Attacks on Israel: The Association of Mortality with a Life-Threatening Stressor," *The Journal of the American Medical Association* 273, 15 (April 1995): 1208–1210.

3. Ibid.

4. S. R. Meisel et al., "Effect of Iraqi Missile War on Incidence of Acute Myocardial Infarction and Sudden Death in Israeli Civilians," *The Lancet* 338, no. 8768 (September 1991): 660–661.

5. Klea Katsouyanni, Manolis Kogevinas, and Mitrios Trichopoulos, "Earthquake-Related Stress and Cardiac Mortality," *International Journal of Epidemiology* 15, no. 3 (December 1985): 326–330.

6. I. Kawachi et al., "Symptoms of Anxiety and Risk of Coronary Heart Disease. The Normative Aging Study," *Circulation* 90 (1994): 2225–2229.

7. A. P. Haines, J. D. Imeson, and T. W. Meade, "Phobic Anxiety and Ischaemic Heart Disease," *British Medical Journal* 295 (August 1987): 297–299.

8. "Can You Be Scared to Death?," *USA Today Magazine,* October 1994.

9. Lana L. Watkins et al., "Phobic Anxiety, Depression, and Risk of Ventricular Arrhythmias in Patients with Coronary Heart Disease," *Psychosomatic Medicine* 68, no. 5 (September/October 2006): 651–656.

10. James L. Januzzi, Jr., et al., "The Influence of Anxiety and Depression on Outcomes of Patients with Coronary Artery Disease," *Archives of Internal Medicine* 160, no. 13 (July 2000): 1913–1921.

11. I. Kawachi et al., "Prospective Study of Phobic Anxiety and Risk of Coronary Heart Disease in Men," *Circulation* 89 (1994): 1992–1997; I. Kawachi et al., "Symptoms of Anxiety and Risk of Coronary Heart Disease. The Normative Aging Study," *Circulation* 90 (1994): 2225–2229; William Coryell, Russell Noyes, and John Clancy, "Excess Mortality in Panic Disorder: A Comparison with Primary Unipolar Depression," *Archives of General Psychiatry* 39, no. 6 (June 1982): 701–703; Coryell, Noyes, and J. D. House, "Mortality among Outpatients with Anxiety Disorders," *American Journal of Psychiatry* 143, no. 4 (April 1986): 508–510.

12. Walter B. Cannon, "'Voodoo' death," *American Anthropologist* 44, no. 2 (April–June 1942):169–181.

13. Curt Richter, "On the Phenomenon of Sudden Death in Animals and Man," *Psychosomatic Medicine* 19, no. 3 (May 1957): 191–198.

14. Murray Esler, et al., "The Peripheral Kinetics of Norepinephrine in Depressive Illness," *Archives of General Psychiatry* 39, no. 3 (March 1982): 295–300.

15. S. B. Manuck et al., "Does Cardiovascular Reactivity to Mental Stress Have Prognostic Value in Postinfarction Patients? A Pilot Study," *Psychosomatic Medicine* 54, no. 1 (January–February 1992): 102–108; D. S. Krantz et al., "Cardiovascular Reactivity and Mental Stress–Induced Myocardial Ischemia in Patients with Coronary Artery Disease," *Psychosomatic Medicine* 53, no. 1 (January–February 1991): 1–12.

16. Kawachi et al., "Symptoms of Anxiety," 2225–2229.

17. Raj Persaud, "Worriers More Prone to Cancer," *New Scientist,* May 28, 2003: http://www.newscientist.com/article/dn3767-worriers-more-prone-to-cancer.html.

18. Alf Forsén, "Psychological Stress as a Risk for Breast Cancer," *Psychotherapy and Psychosomatics* 55, nos. 2–4 (1991): 176–185.

19. Joanna Kruk and Hassan Y. Aboul-Enein, "Psychological Stress and the Risk of Breast Cancer: A Case-Control Study," *Cancer Detection and Prevention* 28, no. 6 (July 2004): 339–408.

20. Kirsi Lillberg et al., "Stressful Life Events and Risk of Breast Cancer in 10,808 Women: A Cohort Study," *American Journal of Epidemiology* 157, no. 5 (2003): 415–423.

21. Felicia D. Roberts et al., "Self-Reported Stress and Risk of Breast Cancer," *Cancer* 77, no. 6 (March 1996): 1089–1093.

22. D. L. Felten et al., "Noradrenergic and Peptidergic Innervation of Lymphoid Tissue," *Journal of Immunology* 135, no. 2 (1985):755s–765s; Y. Shavit et al., "Opioid Peptides Mediate the Suppressive Effect of Stress on Natural Killer Cell Cytotoxicity," *Science* 223, no. 4632 (January 1984): 188–190; Bruce S. Rabin et al., "Bidirectional Interaction Between the Central Nervous System and the Immune System," *Critical Reviews in Immunology* 9, no. 4 (1989): 279–312.

23. Lisa Hurt Kozarovich, "Stress: A Cause of Cancer?," Psych Central: http://psychcentral.com/lib/stress-a-cause-of-cancer/000754.

24. "Stress Weakens the Immune System," *American Psychological Association*, February 23, 2006: http://www.apa.org/research/action/immune.aspx.

25. Robert Ader, David L. Felten, and Nicholas Cohen, eds., *Psychoneuroimmunology* (San Diego: Academic Press, 1991); J. R. Calabrese, M. A. Kling, and P. W. Gold, "Alterations in Immunocompetence During Stress, Bereavement, and Depression: Focus on Neuroendocrine Regulation," *American Journal of Psychiatry* 144, no. 9 (September 1987): 1123–1134; Janice K. Kiecolt-Glaser and Ronald Glaser, "Psychosocial Factors, Stress, Disease, and Immunity," in *Psychoneuroimmunology*, eds. Ader et al. (San Diego: Academic Press, 1991), 849–867.

26. Sheldon Cohen and Gail M. Williamson, "Stress and Infectious Disease in Humans," *Psychological Bulletin* 109, no. 1 (January 1991): 5–24; Mark L. Laudenslager, "Psychosocial Stress and Susceptibility to Infectious Disease," in *Viruses, Immunity, and Mental Disorders*, eds. Edouard Kurstak, Z. J. Lipowski, and P. V. Morozov (New York: Springer, 1987), 391–402.

27. Sheldon Cohen and Tracy B. Herbert, "Health Psychology: Psychological Factors and Physical Disease from the Perspective of Human Psychoneuroimmunology," *Annual Review of Psychology* 47 (February 1996): 113–142; M. Irwin et al., "Life Events, Depressive Symptoms, and Immune Function," *American Journal of Psychiatry* 144, no. 4 (April 1987): 437–441; Steven J. Schleifer et al., "Suppression of Lymphocyte Stimulation Following Bereavement," *The Journal of the American Medical Association* 250, no. 3 (July 1983): 374–377.

28. Martin P. Gallagher et al., "Long-Term Cancer Risk of Immunosuppressive Regimens after Kidney Transplantation," *Journal of the American Society of Nephrology* 21, no. 5 (May 2010): 852–858.

29. J. F. Buell, T. G. Gross, and E. S. Woodle, "Malignancy after Transplantation," *Transplantation* 80, no. 2S (October 2005): S254–S264; Jeremy Chapman and Angela Webster, "Cancer Report," in *ANZDATA Registry 2004 Report* (2004): 99–103; Chapman and Webster, "Cancer after Renal Transplantation: The Next Challenge," *American Journal of Transplantation* 4, no. 6 (June 2004): 841–842.

30. Jørgen H. Olsen et al., "Cancer in the Parents of Children with Cancer," *New England Journal of Medicine* 333 (December 1995): 1594–1599.

31. Jiong Li et al., "Cancer Incidence in Parents Who Lost a Child: A Nationwide Study in Denmark," *Cancer* 95, no. 10 (November 2002): 2237–2242.

32. Anil K. Sood et al., "Adrenergic Modulation of Focal Adhesion Kinase Protects Human Ovarian Cancer Cells from Anoikis," *Journal of Clinical Investigation* 120, no. 5 (May 2010): 1515–1523.

33. Neil M. H. Graham, Robert M. Douglas, and Philip Ryan, "Stress and Acute Respiratory Infection," *American Journal of Epidemiology* 124, no. 3 (1986): 389–401; W. Thomas Boyce et al., "Influence of Life Events and Family Rou-

tines on Childhood Respiratory Tract Illness," *Pediatrics* 60, no. 4 (October 1977): 609–615; Roger J. Meyer and Robert J. Haggerty, "Streptococcal Infections in Families: Factors Altering Individual Susceptibility," *Pediatrics* 29, no. 4 (April 1962): 539–549.

34. Sheldon Cohen, David A. J. Tyrell, and Andrew P. Smith, "Psychological Stress and Susceptibility to the Common Cold," *New England Journal of Medicine* 325, no. 9 (August 1991): 606–612.

35. T. G. Pickering, "Blood Platelets, Stress, and Cardiovascular Disease," *Psychosomatic Medicine* 55, no. 6 (November–December 1993): 483–484; Esther M. Sternberg, "Does Stress Make You Sick and Belief Make You Well? The Science Connecting Body and Mind," *Annals of the New York Academy of Sciences* 917 (January 2000): 1–3.

36. Bert Garssen, "Psychological Factors and Cancer Development: Evidence after 30 Years of Research," *Clinical Psychology Review* 24, no. 3 (July 2004): 315–338; Eric Raible and Allan S. Jaffee, "Work Stress May Be a Determinant of Coronary Heart Disease," *Cardiology Today* 11, no. 3 (March 2008): 33; S. O. Dalton et al., "Mind and Cancer: Do Psychological Factors Cause Cancer?," *European Journal of Cancer* 38, no. 10 (July 2002): 1313–1323; Edna Maria Vissoci Reiche, Sandra Odebrecht Vargas Nunes, and Helena Kaminami Morimoto, "Stress, Depression, the Immune System, and Cancer," *The Lancet Oncology* 5, no. 10 (October 2004): 617–625; Ljudmila Stojanovich and Dragomir Marisavljevich, "Stress as a Trigger of Autoimmune Disease," *Autoimmunity Reviews* 7, no. 3 (January 2008): 209–213; Eva M. Selhub, M.D., "Stress and Distress in Clinical Practice: A Mind-Body Approach," *Nutrition in Clinical Care* 5, no. 4 (August 2002): 182–190.

37. Olivia I. Okereke et al., "High Phobic Anxiety Is Related to Lower Leukocyte Telomere Length in Women," *PLOS ONE* 7, no. 7 (July 2012): e40516.

38. Masahiro Ochi et al., "Effect of Chronic Stress on Gastric Emptying and Plasma Ghrelin Levels in Rats," *Life Sciences* 82, nos. 15–16 (April 2008): 862–868.

39. Jack Sparacino, "Blood Pressure, Stress, and Mental Health," *Nursing Research* 31, no. 2 (March–April 1982): 89–94.

40. Ashley E. Nixon et al., "Can Work Make You Sick? A Meta-Analysis of the Relationships Between Job Stressors and Physical Symptoms," *Work & Stress: An International Journal of Work, Health & Organizations* 25, no. 1 (April 2011): 1–22.

41. Ricard Farré et al., "Critical Role of Stress in Increased Oesophageal Mucosa Permeability and Dilated Intercellular Spaces," *Gut* 56, no. 9 (February 2007): 1191–1197.

42. "Kelly McGonigal: How to Make Stress Your Friend," TED Talk video, 14:28, recorded June 11, 2013, https://www.ted.com/talks/kelly_mcgonigal_how_to_make_stress_your_friend.

43. Lisa M. Schwartz and Steven Woloshin, "Changing Disease Definitions: Implications for Disease Prevalence. Analysis of the Third National Health and Nutrition Examination Survey, 1988–1994," *Effective Clinical Practice* 2, no. 2 (March–April 1999): 76–85.

44. Bart Windrum, "It's Time to Account for Medical Error in 'Top Ten Causes of Death Charts,'" *Journal of Participatory Medicine* 5 (April 2013): http://www.jopm.org/opinion/commentary/2013/04/24/it%E2%80%99s-time-to-account-for-medical-error-in-%E2%80%9Ctop-ten-causes-of-death-charts/.

45. Janet M. Corrigan et al., "To Err Is Human: Building a Safer Health System," *Institute of Medicine of the National Academies* (November 1, 1999): http://www.iom.edu/~/media/Files/Report%20Files/1999/To-Err-is-Human/To%20Err%20is%20Human%201999%20%20report%20brief.pdf.

46. John T. James, "A New, Evidence-Based Estimate of Patient Harms Associated with Hospital Care," *Journal of Patient Safety* 9, no. 3 (September 2013): 122–128.

47. Bill Hendrick, "Americans Worry about Getting Alzheimer's: Survey Reveals Fears About Alzheimer's, Stroke, Heart Disease, and Other Diseases," *WebMD Health News* (February 2011): http://www.webmd.com/alzheimers/news/20110223/americans-worry-about-getting-alzheimers.

48. H. Gilbert Welch and William C. Black, "Overdiagnosis in Cancer," *Journal of the National Cancer Institute* 102, no. 9 (April 2010): 605–613.

49. Heidi D. Nelson et al., "Screening for Breast Cancer: An Update for the U.S. Preventive Services Task Force," *Annals of Internal Medicine* 151, no. 10 (November 2009): 727–W242.

50. H. Gilbert Welch, Lisa M. Schwartz, and Steven Woloshin, *Overdiagnosed: Making People Sick in the Pursuit of Health* (Boston: Beacon Press, 2011), 88.

51. Per-Henrik Zahl, Jan Maehlen, and H. Gilbert Welch, "The Natural History of Invasive Breast Cancers Detected by Screening Mammography," *Archives of Internal Medicine* 168, no. 21 (November 2008): 2311–2316.

52. Ned Calonge et al., "Screening for Breast Cancer: U.S. Preventive Services Task Force Recommendation Statement," *Annals of Internal Medicine* 151, no. 10 (November 2009): 716–726.

53. W. A. Sakr et al., "Age and Racial Distribution of Prostatic Intraepithelial Neoplasia," *European Urology* 30, no. 2 (1996): 138–144.

54. H. Gilbert Welch and Peter C. Albertsen, "Prostate Cancer Diagnosis and Treatment after the Introduction of Prostate-Specific Antigen Screening: 1986–2005," *Journal of the National Cancer Institute* 101, no. 19 (August 2009): 1325–1329.

55. Richard J. Albin, "The Great Prostate Mistake," *The New York Times,* March 9, 2010.

Chapter 3

1. Brian G. Dias and Kerry J. Ressler, "Parental Olfactory Experience Influences Behavior and Neural Structure in Subsequent Generations," *Nature Neuroscience* 17, no. 1 (January 2014): 89–96.

Chapter 6

1. Daniel Gardner, *The Science of Fear* (New York: Plume, 2008), 3.

2. Marc Siegel, "The Irony of Fear," *The Washington Post,* August 30, 2005, http://www.washingtonpost.com/wp-dyn/content/article/2005/08/29/AR2005082901391.html.

3. Gardner, *The Science of Fear,* 8–10.

4. *Psychic Powers,* Mysteries of the Unknown series (Time-Life Books, 1987), 50–53.

Chapter 7

1. "Jill Bolte Taylor: My Stroke of Insight," TED Talk video, 18:19, recorded February 2008, https://www.ted.com/talks/jill_bolte_taylor_s_powerful_stroke_of_insight.

2. Sigmund Freud, "Dreams and the Occult," in *New Introductory Lectures on Psycho-Analysis* (New York: W. W. Norton, 1933), 24.

3. Dean Radin, *The Conscious Universe: The Scientific Truth of Psychic Phenomena* (New York: HarperCollins, 1997), 68–73.

4. Daryl J. Bem and Charles Honorton, "Does Psi Exist? Replicable Evidence for an Anomalous Process of Information Transfer," *Psychological Bulletin* 115, no. 1 (January 1994): 4–18.

5. Ray Hyman, "The Ganzfeld Psi Experiment: A Critical Appraisal," *The Journal of Parapsychology* 49, no. 1 (March 1985): 3–49.

6. Ray Hyman and Charles Honorton, "A Joint Communiqué: The Psi Ganzfeld Controversy," *The Journal of Parapsychology* 50 (December 1986): 351–364.

7. Bem and Honorton, "Does Psi Exist?," 4–18.

8. Julie Milton and Richard Wiseman, "Does Psi Exist? Lack of Replication of an Anomalous Process of Information Transfer," *Psychological Bulletin* 125, no. 4 (July 1999): 387–391.

ACKNOWLEDGMENTS

I have obsessed over what Joyce Carol Oates once said: "I never understand when people make a fuss over me as a writer. I'm just the garden hose that the water sprays through." That's pretty much how I feel about any words that come through me. What I know for sure is that I'd just be a messy, clogged, and kinked garden hose if it weren't for the people who helped me let the water spray through. If this book helps anyone heal, it's only because of some miraculous combination of the grace of God and those people who made it possible. Without their hand-holding and hose-unkinking, I simply could not have written it.

I must say this book became a beast I had no idea would fight me so fiercely, surely because my garden hose was wound so tight. As I got started, my cognitive mind researched and easefully wrote Part One of this book before the rest of me realized, "Oh crikey! I've just scared them more!" and was stunned silent—for two years. Then, in January 2014, with only three months until my book was due, I wound up teaching a teleclass series with my longtime friend and mentor Rachel Naomi Remen, M.D., who graciously wrote the foreword for this book. For two months, I sat at Rachel's famous Kitchen Table every day and was moved, time and time again, to tears. About a month into our daily meetings, Rachel said, "Lissa, do you know why I am teaching Medicine for the Soul with you?" I had felt humbled and inadequate when she agreed to teach with me. I assumed she had done it so we could generate revenue to help support her nonprofit work. She shook her head and smiled with so much love. She told me she had done it so we could help grow each other's souls.

I now suspect that the purposeful universe arranged for Rachel and me to sit side by side for two months so this book could be born. All I did was show up at my computer with willing hands, while something much larger than me flowed through my fingers, while Rachel held the possibility of this book gently, like she was tending a rosebud. Words cannot begin to express my gratitude to you, Rachel. When I was solidly stuck in my victim role, you loved me back to wholeness. Your presence in my life can only be described as the unearned blessing of *grace.* You are my family, and I appreciate you so much.

Infinite thanks also to Martha Beck, who once told me she would "hold the plane" for me when I was doubting my own journey through fear. Not understanding what she meant, I raised an eyebrow. Martha said, "You know how sometimes you're dashing through the airport, with your bags banging into everything, rushing to try to make your flight. But then you remember that your friend is already on the plane, and she can tell the pilot, 'Wait! Hold the plane! My friend is coming!'" When I started writing *The Fear Cure,* I had no faith that I would ever make it to the plane you were already on, Martha, but knowing that you believed I would get there in time somehow made it possible. I borrowed your faith when I didn't have enough of my own. My gratitude for you is a waterfall that will never stop flowing. Thank you for introducing me to magic, tirelessly researching the mystical, normalizing my "crazy" experiences, and always leaving me laughing at the marvel of it all.

Much of the work of unclogging my garden hose came through Tosha Silver, who lovingly and fiercely held me accountable to staying aligned with what I was writing about and reminded me often who was really doing the writing. Many times I forgot and strayed out of alignment, and—bless your heart, Tosha—you never let me get away with straying far off course. Every time I thought I finally understood what you were teaching, my Small Self would find a new sneaky way to disguise itself and try to grab the wheel of Lissa. Thank God you were never fooled, and each time you steered me gently back to the truth. Meeting you has been a miracle.

If this book had a scenic backdrop, it would be the snowy mountains of Lake Tahoe, where I spent many hours sitting in a meadow while hashing out the content for this book with my soul twin Dennis Couwenberg, who was brave enough to go deep into the shadows with me as we took on the challenge of stripping back the onion layers of ego to illuminate our darkest fears together. Dennis, your willingness to examine your own relationship with fear—and to let me share your stories publicly—enriched this book beyond measure. You have been such an inspiration to me. As you sat there on that rollercoaster, strapped yourself into that harness to brave the ropes course, took on the inner journey of your silent retreat with Adyashanti, showed up for us both with Rose, faced your resistance by hiking up into the Andes, risked everything by leaving your stable career behind, and took on the demons of The General with the "game on" playfulness of your Magical Child, you demonstrated to me what it means to live a life of raw courage. Every time I think you've hit the end of what you're willing to take on, you go further. And because you fill the journey to enlightenment with so much playfulness, I can't resist coming with you. I will be forever grateful that you blew into my life, bringing with you a glimpse of freedom. I never wanted to do my work in this world alone, and now that I've found you, I trust that whatever we are meant to explore together in this world will unfold perfectly. When I think of getting up on stage with you beside me, I get goose bumps and feel like anything is possible. Thank you for reminding me who I am, why I'm here, and how unconditional love and total freedom really can coexist.

To April Sweazy, whom I dedicated this book to, when I see you every morning with your tousled hair and sleepy eyes, I pinch myself and laugh at the Universe's wild sense of humor. I still remember you flying across the country to do a session with me all those years ago, when I had no idea what I was doing and you had no idea why you were flying to California to do a coaching session with some stranger. All I can say is that it's a good thing Someone is orchestrating life way better than we ever could have! It's a daily joy to have you as part of the family and to witness the courage you continue to demonstrate more and more all the time. Thank you for always having my back, for being a sounding board as I struggled through this book, for loving me unconditionally, for teaching me what real healing means, and for bravely adopting us as your family. I am grateful.

A special shout-out also goes to Sarah Drew, who steadfastly, with zero judgment, journeyed beside me as I struggled on the spiritual path. I once heard that when a soul has chosen to come to earth in a challenging human role, her spirit guide may choose to incarnate with her, in order to ease the journey and guide her through in human form. When I heard that, I instantly knew that if this was true, Sarah was the spirit guide who came here, like Mother Gaia herself, to wrap me in her expansive arms, engulf me in the feminine, and make it all okay. Thank you, Sarah, for being the best friend anyone could ever have.

Thank you, Anne Davin, for honing in like a laser on Truth and inviting me to see it through the lens of your brilliant perspective. Thank you also for all that you do with the business to amplify what we teach, ground it, deepen it, and lift it up. I'm also grateful to Bruce Cryer, who danced with me for a year before we ever knew each other's names and who now runs my business, bringing to it the most gentle presence. Running this business with you is a joy. Thank you also to Pearl Roth and Beth Elliott, without whom none of my work would be possible. Without your tireless and often thankless dedication, we wouldn't be gathering souls in communion the way we do. Thank you also to Bridgette Boudreau, whose work as the CEO of Martha Beck, Inc., and whose genuine friendship and guidance has steered me like a beacon in a business full of land mines.

Huge gratitude also goes to my best girlfriends Cari Hernandez, Rebecca Bass, Elisabeth Manning, Christine Hassler, Melanie Bates, Linda Rose, Rachel Carlton Abrams, Amy Ahlers, Tricia Barrett, Sera Beak, Katsy Johnson, Maggie Varadhan, Kira Siebert, and Kris Carr, who have unconditionally loved and accepted me and my Small Self for many years, always standing for my soul while gently comforting the scared, small parts of me that have resisted my own growth. You have been steadfast in your support of me, and I am ever grateful.

I am also immensely grateful to the Divine men in my life—Jon Rasmussen, Nicholas Wilton, Fred Kraziese, Steve Sisgold, Chris Guillebeau, Rafael Bejarano, Nick Polizzi, Scott Dinsmore, Larry Dossey, Jonathan Fields, and Ken Jaques. Without the masculine arms within which you have all held me, I wouldn't have been able to let go on the dance floor of life the way I do.

A special thanks to Barbara Stanny, who gifted me with the use of her Lake Tahoe chalet, where most of this book was birthed. Thank you to the late Elizabeth Lloyd Mayer ("Lisby"), whose book research and book *Extraordinary Knowing* deeply influenced this book. Thank you also to Betsy Rapaport, who helped finish Lisby's book after Lisby died. Sometimes it takes one scientist speaking to another to crack the shell of ego that makes us lose the eyes to see.

Thank you also to my family—Siena Klein, Matt Klein, Trish Rankin, Chris Rankin, Keli Rankin, and, if he were still with us, Dave Rankin. I know this journey I've been on has been challenging for all of us. When we wake up and start to question the unconscious agreements we've made with our families and dismantle codependence, it can easily be mistaken for rejection, when really, it's a whole new level of healthy love. Thank you for your patience with me, and please know that I love you all beyond measure and am infinitely grateful I hit the jackpot of being born a Rankin in this lifetime.

Thank you to all of the physicians and health care providers in the Whole Health Medicine Institute. Knowing you are in the world, acting as ambassadors for the work presented in my books, brings immeasurable peace to my heart, reminding me that it really does take a village. Bless you for being my village and making it possible for me to do the work I do with so much pleasure! I love you all and am unspeakably grateful.

And of course, to everyone at Hay House, without whom this book would never have come into being, enormous thanks, especially to Reid Tracy, Louise Hay, Patty Gift, Anne Barthel, Sally Mason, Richelle Zizian, and Lindsay McGinty, for supporting me fiercely as I took on the behemoth of this book. I'm also very grateful to Bob Marty, who produced my national public television special about *The Fear Cure*. And savoring one of my biggest appreciations last, I'm especially grateful to my literary agent and dearest friend, Michele Martin, who walked with me to the edge of crazy and back, without ever once making me worry that she wouldn't be certain to come all the way with me, wherever I dared to go. Michele, you have lived this book with me, championing it (and my role as its spokesperson) when I doubted it all and was ready to throw in the towel. Were it not for you, *The Fear Cure* would not exist as anything other than scribbles on napkins and meaningless mumbo-jumbo in a dozen Word documents I might never have been brave enough to tackle. It really does take a village to write a book like this, and I have been incredibly blessed with a community of loving, supportive fellow villagers. In an industry that tends to try to keep authors in safe, predictable boxes, it has been an enormous blessing to feel so courageously supported by all involved in the creation and distribution of this message as I pushed the envelope of what "medicine" really can be.

Because of everyone I've mentioned here—and those I haven't mentioned by name who have also blessed me and this book (you know who you are, beloveds!)—I have learned what love really is. Byron Katie says that personalities can't love. They just want something. But once fear moves to the side, a new kind of love can step in. I now define love this way: *Love is gently pushing the leading edge of soul growth (for yourself and another) while patiently comforting the lagging edge of the Small Self (for yourself and another).* It takes everything I have to accept that I might actually be worthy of such an expansive love. The way I see it, the Universe sent some of the most enlightened people on the planet to love me into alignment and help me write this book. It almost feels too good to be true, until I breathe . . . and know that love is who we are, and we are all just remembering what has been true all along.

The ultimate acknowledgment goes to that which lives in me and in you, surrounding us and animating All That Is, that which did the actual writing of this book and breathes life force into each of us as the unique expression of the Infinite. What a blessing. I am grateful grateful grateful.

ABOUT THE AUTHOR

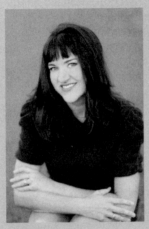 **Dr Lissa Rankin** author of the *New York Times* bestseller *Mind Over Medicine*, is a physician, author speaker, and founder of the Whole Health Medicine Institute, a training programme for physicians and other health care providers. Passionate about what makes people healthy and what predisposes them to illness, she studies how healers might better care for patients and how patients might better care for themselves. She is on a mission to heal health care, help patients play a more active role in healing themselves, learn from indigenous cultures about anomalous forms of healing and encourage the health care industry to embrace and facilitate, rather than resist, such miracles. She is also passionate about how spiritual growth translates into physical healing and how awakening collective consciousness heals us all.

www.lissarankin.com

Hay House Titles of Related Interest

YOU CAN HEAL YOUR LIFE, the movie, starring Louise Hay & Friends
(available as a 1-DVD programme and an expanded 2-DVD set)
Watch the trailer at: www.LouiseHayMovie.com

THE SHIFT, the movie,
starring Dr Wayne W. Dyer
(available as a 1-DVD programme and an expanded 2-DVD set)
Watch the trailer at: www.DyerMovie.com

———

ALL IS WELL: Heal Your Body with Medicine, Affirmations and Intuition,
by Louise Hay and Mona Lisa Schulz MD PhD

DAILY LOVE: Growing into Grace, by Mastin Kipp

DEFY GRAVITY: Healing Beyond the Bounds of Reason, by Caroline Myss

LIFE'S OPERATING MANUAL: With the Fear and Truth Dialogues,
by Tom Shadyac

*LOVE YOUR ENEMIES: How to Break the Anger Habit & Be a Whole Lot
Happier,* by Sharon Salzberg and Robert Thurman

All of the above are available at your local bookstore,
or may be ordered by contacting Hay House.

———